A Text Book of Pharmaceutics for I Year Diploma in Pharmacy

Dr. Sowjanya Gurugubelli
Mr. Prakash Nathaniel Kumar Sarella
Mr. Shaikh Samir Karim Karim
Mrs. Prathyusha Vuddanda
Mrs. Vijayalakshmi M K
Mrs. Jhansipriya Marabathuni V
Mrs. Vinny Therissa Mangam
Mrs. Chollangi Bharghavi
Dr. Bala Venkata Sivaram Nallamolu
Mr. Anilkumar Vadaga

ISBN: 9788197973178

Editors

Dr. Sowjanya Gurugubelli

Mrs. Jhansipriya Marabathuni V

Mr. Prakash Nathaniel Kumar Sarella

Mrs. Vinny Therissa Mangam

Mr. Shaikh Samir Karim Karim

Mrs. Chollangi Bharghavi

Mrs. Prathyusha Vuddanda

Dr. Bala Venkata Sivaram Nallamolu

Mrs. Vijayalakshmi M K

Mr. Anilkumar Vadaga

First Edition: 2024
ISBN: 9788197973178

Maximum Retail Price: Rs. 500/- (Inclusive of all taxes)

Published by ThinkPlus Pharma Publications,
9-15/1, Indrapalem, Kakinada, AP-533006, India.
Website: www.books.jopir.in

Printed at Tarangini Printing Works, Subhadra Arcade, Bhanugudi, Kakinada, AP-533003, India.

DEDICATION

We dedicate this textbook to the future generations of pharmacists who are taking their first steps into the fascinating world of pharmaceutics. May this work inspire and guide you through your educational journey and beyond. We also dedicate this book to our students, past and present, whose curiosity and enthusiasm have continually motivated us to strive for excellence in pharmacy education. Finally, we extend this dedication to all healthcare professionals who tirelessly work to improve patient care and advance the field of pharmacy.

CONTENTS

ACKNOWLEDGMENTS

We, the authors, express our sincere gratitude to the numerous individuals and institutions that have supported us throughout the creation of this textbook. Our deepest thanks go to our colleagues and mentors in the pharmaceutical sciences, whose expertise and guidance have been instrumental in shaping this comprehensive work. We are profoundly grateful to the faculty and staff of various Diploma in Pharmacy programs, whose valuable feedback and suggestions have significantly enhanced the content and structure of this book. We extend our appreciation to the pharmaceutical industry professionals and researchers whose groundbreaking work has informed and enriched our content. Our heartfelt thanks go to our families for their unwavering support and understanding during the writing process. Lastly, we acknowledge the diligent efforts of our publishing team, whose expertise has been crucial in bringing this collaborative project to fruition.

CHAPTER 1

HISTORICAL BACKGROUND AND DEVELOPMENT OF PROFESSION OF PHARMACY

Author

Dr. Chennupati V Suresh

Professor, Nalanda College of Pharmacy,

Nalgonda, Telangana State, India

Abstract

The profession of pharmacy has evolved significantly from its ancient roots to its current status as an integral part of modern healthcare. Early civilizations recognized the medicinal properties of plants, leading to the development of traditional healing practices. The emergence of apothecaries in medieval Europe marked a crucial step towards the formalization of pharmacy as a distinct profession. The Renaissance period saw advancements in chemical and botanical knowledge, contributing to the expansion of the pharmacist's role. The 18th and 19th centuries witnessed the isolation of active compounds from plants and the birth of synthetic drug manufacturing, revolutionizing pharmaceutical practice. The 20th century brought about significant changes, including the industrialization of drug production, the development of new dosage forms, and the expansion of clinical pharmacy services. Today, pharmacists play diverse roles in healthcare, from medication management to patient counseling and public health initiatives. The profession continues to adapt to technological advancements, evolving healthcare needs, and the increasing complexity of drug therapies, emphasizing the importance of lifelong learning and interprofessional collaboration in modern pharmacy practice.

Keywords: *Apothecary, Drug discovery, Professional evolution, Healthcare, Pharmaceutical science, Clinical pharmacy*

Learning Objectives

After completion of the chapter, the student should be able to:

- Understand the evolution of pharmacy as a profession from ancient times to the present day.
- Identify key milestones and influential figures in the history of pharmacy.
- Explain the transition from traditional apothecaries to modern pharmaceutical practices.
- Describe the development of pharmacology and its impact on the pharmacy profession.
- Discuss the role of pharmacy in healthcare systems throughout history.
- Analyze the changing responsibilities and scope of practice for pharmacists over time.
- Evaluate the impact of technological advancements on the pharmacy profession.

INTRODUCTION TO PHARMACEUTICS

Pharmaceutics: Pharmaceutics is a fundamental discipline within pharmacy that focuses on the transformation of new chemical entities (NCEs) or existing drugs into safe and effective medications for patient use. This field encompasses the science of dosage form design, which is crucial for optimizing drug delivery and therapeutic outcomes.

Drug

The term "drug" originates from the French word 'drogue', meaning herb, reflecting the historical roots of pharmacy in natural remedies. In modern pharmacology, a drug is defined as any agent used in the treatment, prevention, mitigation, cure, or diagnosis of diseases or disorders in humans or animals. Drugs utilized in contemporary medical practice are either synthetic or derived from natural sources, including vegetable, animal, or mineral origins.

Drug sources have diversified significantly over time. While many pharmaceuticals still originate from natural sources, such as plants (e.g., morphine from Papaver somniferum), animals (e.g., heparin from porcine intestinal mucosa), or minerals (e.g., calcium carbonate), an increasing number are synthetic or semi-synthetic. Advances in medicinal chemistry and biotechnology have led to the development of novel drug entities and biologics, expanding the therapeutic arsenal available to healthcare professionals.

Dosage form

A dosage form is the final, administrable presentation of a drug, created by combining the active pharmaceutical ingredient (API) with non-drug components known as excipients or additives. Excipients encompass a wide range of substances, including binders, disintegrants, lubricants, preservatives, flavoring agents, and coloring agents. The selection and proportion of these ingredients are critical in determining the physicochemical properties, stability, and therapeutic efficacy of the final dosage form

The desirable properties of dosage forms are:

1. It should be convenient to handle, use and store. For better compliance it should not disturb his routine lifestyle as far as possible and should be acceptable aesthetically, organoleptically, therapeutically and from economic standpoint.

2. It should be stable during storage and use. During storage the physical, chemical and therapeutic integrity of

the dosage form should be maintained by assuring freedom from interaction between components, with packaging materials and environmental factors (heat, humidity, oxygen, light). It should also withstand mechanical shock during transportation. The dosage form should retain its shape, size, appearance, taste, flavor and therapeutic effect during the stipulated half life.

3. The dosage form should be represented in different dosage form strengths providing flexibility of dose to suit different age groups (50, 100,200mg etc)

4. It should provide anticipated therapeutic effect. The extent and pattern of drug release from the dosage form should be predictable.

5. It should protect the drug substance and conceal the disagreeable taste or odour.

6. It should be economical and presentation should be elegant.

7. Finally it should permit easy identification through distinct colour, shape or identification marking.

Classification of Dosage forms:

According to physical state: Solid, semi solid, liquid, gaseous.

Route of administration: Oral. Parenteral, rectal, nasal

Site of application: Skin, eye, tooth, hand, foot, hair, nose etc

Use: External, Internal

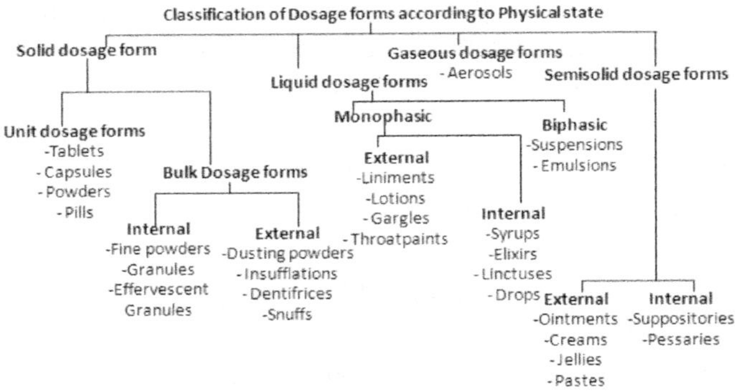

Figure: Classification of dosage forms according to physical state

Definitions

Tablets: Tablets are solid unit dosage forms containing one or more medicaments, with or without appropriate excipients. They are primarily manufactured through compression, although molding techniques may also be employed in some cases. While tablets are predominantly designed for oral administration, they can be formulated for other routes as well. The compression process involves the application of high pressure to a powder mixture, resulting in a coherent, uniform, and stable product. Tablets offer several advantages, including precise dosing, ease of administration, and improved stability compared to liquid formulations. They can be formulated to provide immediate release, modified release, or targeted delivery of the active ingredient(s). Common examples include Aminophylline tablets for bronchodilation, Chloroquine sulphate tablets for malaria treatment, and Paracetamol tablets for pain relief and fever reduction. The formulation of tablets typically includes the active pharmaceutical ingredient(s) (APIs), diluents (e.g., lactose, microcrystalline cellulose), binders (e.g., povidone, hydroxypropyl methylcellulose), disintegrants (e.g., croscarmellose sodium, sodium starch glycolate), lubricants (e.g., magnesium stearate), and sometimes other functional excipients such as glidants or colorants

Capsules: Capsules are solid dosage forms in which the medicament is enclosed within a soluble container or shell, typically made of gelatin. This shell serves to mask the taste of the drug and facilitate swallowing. Capsules are classified into two main types: hard gelatin capsules and soft gelatin capsules.

Hard gelatin capsules consist of two parts - a body and a cap - and are primarily used for encapsulating solid or semi-solid formulations. They are filled with powders, granules, or pellets containing the active ingredient(s) and necessary excipients. Examples include Amoxicillin capsules for bacterial infections and Ampicillin capsules for various infectious diseases. Soft gelatin capsules, also known as softgels, are one-piece capsules that can encapsulate liquids, semi-solids, or solids. They are particularly useful for poorly water-soluble drugs or those that require protection from oxidation. Soft gelatin capsules are often used for vitamins, minerals, and some antibiotics.

Powders: Powders represent a versatile solid dosage form that can be used for both internal (oral) and external applications. Oral powders are designed for internal use and may be administered directly or reconstituted with water before ingestion. These can be simple (containing a single active ingredient) or compound (containing multiple active ingredients). Examples include Compound rhubarb powder, used as a laxative, and Compound sodium chloride and dextrose oral powder, used for oral rehydration therapy. Dusting powders, on the other hand, are intended for external use and are applied topically to the skin. They often contain ingredients like talc, zinc oxide, or starch and may be medicated or non-medicated. Talc dusting powder is a common example, used to absorb moisture and reduce friction on the skin.

Pills: Pills are an antiquated solid dosage form that predates tablets in the evolution of unit dosage forms. They were developed to address the inconvenience associated with administering loose powders. Pills are spherical in shape, which was thought to facilitate swallowing. The manufacturing process typically involved mixing the medicinal powder with a suitable excipient to form a plastic mass, which was then rolled into a cylinder and divided into sections of equal weight. These sections were then rolled between the fingers to produce spherical pills.

While pills were once a popular dosage form, they have largely been supplanted by tablets and capsules in modern pharmaceutical practice. This is due to several factors, including:

- Difficulty in achieving content uniformity
- Lack of precision in dosing
- Challenges in large-scale manufacturing
- Potential for variability in disintegration and dissolution.

Granules: Granules are a solid dosage form of medicaments that serve as an intermediate product in tablet manufacturing or as a final dosage form for direct administration. The process of granulation involves mixing powdered drug(s) with excipients, including sweetening, flavoring, and coloring agents, to improve taste and appearance. A granulating agent, typically a liquid binder, is added to moisten the powder mixture and facilitate particle agglomeration.

The wet mass is then passed through a sieve to create

uniformly sized granules, which are subsequently dried at a controlled temperature, often around 60°C. This drying process is crucial to remove excess moisture and ensure stability. Granules are commonly supplied in glass containers with instructions for the patient to reconstitute them with freshly boiled and cooled water, creating a liquid preparation at the time of use.

Granules offer several advantages:

- Improved flow properties compared to powders
- Enhanced content uniformity
- Reduced dust formation during handling
- Increased stability and shelf life
- Potential for controlled release formulations.

Effervescent Granules: Effervescent Granules are a specialized solid dosage form designed for internal use. They typically contain a combination of acids (such as citric acid and tartaric acid) and a carbonate or bicarbonate salt (usually sodium bicarbonate), along with the active medicament. A sweetening agent like saccharin or sucrose may be added to improve palatability

$$3NaHCO_3 + C_6H_8O_7.H_2O \xrightarrow{\Delta} C_6H_5Na_3O_7 + 3CO_2 + 3H_2O$$
$$2NaHCO_3 + C_4H_6O_6 \xrightarrow{\Delta} C_4H_4Na_2O_6 + 2CO_2 + 2H_2O$$

The effervescent reaction occurs when these granules are added to water. This reaction produces carbon dioxide gas, creating a pleasant, fizzy sensation and often enhancing the dissolution of the active ingredient. Effervescent granules are commonly used for:

- Antacid preparations
- Analgesics and antipyretics
- Vitamin and mineral supplements
- Oral rehydration therapies

The effervescence can mask unpleasant tastes, improve dissolution rates, and potentially enhance absorption of certain drugs. Patients are typically instructed to consume the preparation while effervescing or immediately afterward for optimal effect

Dusting powders: Dusting Powders are topical formulations intended for external application to the skin. They are typically composed of two or more finely divided, inert ingredients such as starch, kaolin, talc, or zinc oxide. The fine particle size is crucial for their effectiveness and to minimize potential skin irritation. To ensure homogeneity and appropriate particle size, these powders are often passed through a fine mesh sieve (e.g., sieve no. 120).

Dusting powders can be categorized as medicated or non-medicated:

- Medicated dusting powders contain active pharmaceutical ingredients for specific therapeutic effects.
- Non-medicated dusting powders primarily serve protective or cosmetic purposes.

The functions of dusting powders include:

- Antiseptic: To prevent or treat minor skin infections
- Antipruritic: To relieve itching
- Astringent: To constrict body tissues
- Antiperspirant: To reduce sweating
- Absorbent: To absorb excess moisture
- Protective: To create a barrier on the skin
- Lubricant: To reduce friction between skin surfaces

It's important to note that dusting powders should not be applied to open wounds or raw surfaces due to the risk of granuloma formation or other complications. Examples include dicophane dusting powder (an insecticide), zinc and salicylic acid dusting powder (for fungal infections), and zinc, starch and talc dusting powder (for general skin protection).

Insufflations: Insufflations are finely divided powder formulations designed for introduction into body cavities such as the ears, nose, tooth sockets, or vagina. They are administered using a specialized device called an insufflator, which helps deliver the powder to areas that would be difficult to reach directly.

The primary advantages of insufflations include:

- Targeted delivery to specific body cavities
- Potential for both local and systemic effects (particularly with intranasal administration)
- Improved residence time compared to liquid formulations

However, traditional insufflators have some drawbacks:

- Difficulty in regulating uniform dose delivery
- Potential for irritation due to powder inhalation
- Limited patient acceptability

To address these limitations, modern pharmaceutical technology has largely replaced traditional insufflators with more advanced delivery systems, such as metered-dose inhalers and nasal sprays. These newer formats offer several improvements:

- More precise dose control
- Reduced risk of inhalation and associated irritation
- Improved ease of use and patient compliance
- Better stability and shelf life.

Dentifrices: Dentifrices are oral hygiene products designed to maintain dental health and cleanliness. These preparations, available primarily as tooth powders and pastes, serve multiple functions in oral care. They aid in cleaning tooth surfaces, removing plaque and food debris, preventing dental caries, and freshening breath. The composition of dentifrices is complex, typically including cleaning agents such as soaps or detergents, with sodium lauryl sulfate being a common choice. These surfactants help dislodge and remove plaque and food particles from the teeth. To enhance mechanical cleaning without damaging tooth enamel, dentifrices incorporate mild abrasives. Substances like calcium carbonate, silica, or aluminum hydroxide serve this purpose effectively. A crucial component in modern dentifrices is the anti-cariogenic agent, most commonly a fluoride compound such as sodium fluoride or stannous fluoride. These fluoride compounds play a vital role in preventing tooth decay by promoting the remineralization of tooth enamel. The formulation of dentifrices also includes humectants, such as glycerin or sorbitol, which prevent the product from drying out and maintain its consistency. Flavoring agents are added to improve taste and user acceptance, while preservatives extend shelf life and prevent microbial growth. In paste formulations, thickening agents are incorporated to achieve the desired consistency. Contemporary dentifrices often feature additional active ingredients to address specific oral health concerns. These may include desensitizing agents like potassium nitrate for sensitive teeth, whitening agents such as hydrogen peroxide, tartar control agents like pyrophosphates, and antimicrobial agents such as triclosan or chlorhexidine for enhanced oral hygiene.

Snuffs: Snuffs represent a unique solid dosage form of medicaments designed for nasal inhalation. These finely divided powder preparations are formulated to deliver therapeutic agents directly to the nasal mucosa, potentially eliciting both local and systemic effects. Traditionally, snuffs have been employed for their antiseptic action in combating nasal infections, bronchodilatory effects to alleviate respiratory congestion, and decongestant properties to reduce nasal swelling and mucus production. The example of

Maxeran, a metoclopramide snuff, illustrates an innovative approach to drug delivery. Metoclopramide, typically used as an antiemetic and prokinetic agent, is formulated as a nasal snuff, suggesting potential exploration of alternative administration routes for systemic effects. The formulation of snuffs requires careful consideration of particle size to ensure effective deposition in the nasal cavity while minimizing irritation to the nasal mucosa. Stability of the active ingredient and ease of administration are also crucial factors in snuff development. It is worth noting that the use of snuffs has declined in modern pharmaceutical practice, largely supplanted by nasal sprays and other more controlled delivery systems that offer improved dosing accuracy and patient acceptance

Liniments: Liniments are liquid or semi-liquid preparations intended for topical application to the skin. These formulations are designed to be applied with friction or rubbing, which enhances the absorption of active ingredients and promotes local therapeutic effects. Liniments can be formulated as alcoholic or oily solutions, or as emulsions, each type offering specific benefits depending on the intended use and active ingredients. The application of liniments through massage or rubbing not only aids in the absorption of active compounds but also provides a therapeutic effect through the physical act of massage itself. This dual action makes liniments particularly useful for treating muscle pain, stiffness, and other musculoskeletal discomforts. To ensure proper use and safety, liniments are typically dispensed in colored, fluted bottles, distinguishing them from preparations meant for internal use. Clear labeling instructions, such as "FOR EXTERNAL USE ONLY" and "SHAKE THE BOTTLE BEFORE USE," are crucial to prevent misuse and ensure optimal efficacy. Common examples of liniments include soap liniment, which contains soap, camphor, and alcohol, and is often used for muscle pain and stiffness. Another example is white liniment, an emulsion containing turpentine, acetic acid, and egg, which acts as a counterirritant. The active ingredients in liniments can vary widely, including analgesics like methyl salicylate, counterirritants such as capsaicin, or anti-inflammatory agents like diclofenac.

Table: Lotions Vs Liniments

Characteristic	Lotions	Liniments
Consistency	Liquid, often thinner	Liquid to semi-liquid, often thicker
Application method	Applied without friction	Applied with rubbing or massage
Base	Often water-based	Often alcohol or oil-based
Primary purpose	Soothing, cooling, moisturizing	Pain relief, muscle relaxation
Absorption	Generally quick absorption	Slower absorption, aided by friction
Common ingredients	Water, glycerin, emollients	Alcohol, oils, counterirritants
Skin penetration	Typically superficial	Often deeper penetration
Duration of effect	Generally shorter-lasting	Often longer-lasting
Common uses	Skin hydration, minor skin issues	Muscle aches, joint pain

Lotions: Lotions represent another category of topical

preparations, distinct from liniments in their application method and composition. These liquid preparations are intended for external application to the skin without friction. Lotions can exist as monophasic (single-phase) or biphasic (two-phase) systems, typically formulated as liquid suspensions or dispersions. The composition of lotions often includes alcohol or glycerin, each serving specific purposes. Alcohol provides a cooling sensation upon application and promotes quick drying, while glycerin helps maintain skin moisture for an extended period. This combination of ingredients allows lotions to provide various local actions such as cooling, soothing, protecting, or exerting antiseptic effects. Like liniments, lotions are dispensed in colored, fluted bottles to differentiate them from internal use preparations, and they carry similar labeling requirements for safety. The instruction to shake the bottle before use is particularly important for biphasic lotions to ensure proper mixing of the ingredients before application.

Calamine lotion, containing calamine and zinc oxide, is a classic example used for soothing itchy or irritated skin. Another common formulation is salicylic acid lotion, which finds use in treating acne or as a keratolytic agent. The versatility of lotions extends to various dermatological applications, including moisturizing dry skin, treating skin conditions like eczema or psoriasis, providing sun protection, and even serving as insect repellents. The liquid nature of lotions facilitates easy spreading over large areas of skin and promotes quick absorption. This characteristic makes lotions particularly suitable for treating extensive skin surfaces or for frequent application.

Gargles: Gargles are aqueous solutions specifically formulated for oral and throat care. These preparations are designed to combat throat infections and provide relief from associated symptoms. Typically supplied in concentrated form, gargles require dilution with warm water before use, enhancing their efficacy and ensuring patient comfort. The act of gargling involves bringing the solution into close contact with the mucous membranes of the throat, allowing it to remain there momentarily before expulsion. This process facilitates the delivery of active ingredients to the affected area, promoting therapeutic effects. Some gargles, particularly those containing analgesics like aspirin, may be swallowed after use, providing both local and systemic benefits. The dual action of these preparations can be especially beneficial in managing throat pain and inflammation. To ensure proper identification and use, gargles are typically dispensed in white fluted bottles, distinguishing them from other oral preparations.

Mouthwashes: Mouthwashes, while similar to gargles in their aqueous nature, serve a broader range of purposes in oral hygiene. These concentrated solutions are formulated with pleasant tastes and flavors to encourage regular use. Their functions extend beyond mere refreshment, often including deodorizing and antiseptic properties. Medicated mouthwashes may incorporate various active ingredients such as astringents, antibacterial agents, or protein precipitants, each targeting specific oral health concerns. Like gargles, mouthwashes are generally diluted with warm water before use. They are designed to be swished around the oral cavity, coming into contact with the teeth, gums, and mucous membranes. This widespread application allows for comprehensive oral care. Examples of mouthwashes include compound sodium chloride and zinc sulphate mouthwash, and zinc chloride mouthwash, each offering unique benefits for oral health.

Sprays: Sprays represent a versatile dosage form for delivering medicaments to the nose or throat. These liquid preparations can be formulated with aqueous, alcoholic, or glycerin-containing vehicles, allowing for customization based on the active ingredients and intended use. The use of atomizers or nebulizers for application ensures fine dispersion of the medication, promoting even distribution and absorption across the target tissues. Examples of medicinal sprays include compound adrenaline and atropine spray, used for nasal decongestion and to reduce secretions, and isoprenaline spray, which can be employed in the management of asthma symptoms. The spray format allows for precise, localized delivery of these potent medications, minimizing systemic exposure and potential side effects

Collodions: Collodions are unique liquid preparations designed for external application to the skin. Their primary function is to form a protective film over small cuts, abrasions, or areas requiring prolonged contact with a medicament. The distinctive feature of collodions is their volatile vehicle, which evaporates upon application, leaving behind a flexible, adherent film that acts as a barrier and delivery system for active ingredients. The composition of flexible collodion typically includes pyroxylon as the film-forming agent, castor oil for flexibility, and a mixture of alcohol and solvent ether as the vehicle. This formulation strikes a balance between protective properties and comfort, allowing the film to move with the skin without cracking or peeling. Collodions are usually applied using a brush or rod, allowing for precise application to small areas. This method of application, combined with the quick-drying nature of the preparation, makes collodions particularly useful for treating minor skin injuries or delivering medications to specific skin sites. The resulting film not only protects the area from external contaminants but also maintains close contact between the active ingredients and the skin, potentially enhancing therapeutic efficacy.

Spirits: Spirits are liquid pharmaceutical preparations that utilize alcohol as the primary solvent, typically at a concentration of 90 percent. This high alcohol content serves multiple purposes in the formulation. Firstly, it acts as an excellent solvent for many medicinal compounds, ensuring their complete dissolution and uniform distribution throughout the preparation. Secondly, the high alcohol concentration provides preservative properties, inhibiting microbial growth and extending the shelf life of the product. Examples of spirits include chloroform spirit, lemon spirit, and compound orange spirit. These preparations often combine the medicinal properties of their active ingredients with the aromatic qualities of essential oils or other flavoring agents. For instance, chloroform spirit may be used for its mild analgesic and antispasmodic properties, while lemon and orange spirits can serve as flavoring agents in other pharmaceutical preparations or as aromatic stimulants. The high alcohol content of spirits also allows for rapid absorption of the active ingredients when administered, making them particularly useful for certain types of medications that require quick onset of action. However, this high alcohol concentration also necessitates careful consideration of dosing and potential interactions with other medications or medical conditions.

Throat paints: Throat paints represent a specialized category of viscous liquid preparations designed specifically for treating mouth and throat infections. These formulations are characterized by their thick consistency, which allows them to adhere to the mucous membranes of the oral and pharyngeal regions for extended periods. This prolonged contact time enhances the therapeutic effect of the active ingredients. Glycerin is frequently employed as a base in throat paints due to its multiple beneficial properties. Its viscous nature ensures that the preparation clings to the treated area, resisting rapid washout by saliva. Additionally, glycerin's hygroscopic properties help to maintain moisture in the treated tissues, potentially soothing irritation. The agreeable taste of glycerin also improves patient acceptability, which is particularly important for oral preparations. Examples of throat paints include boroglycerin, which combines the antimicrobial properties of boric acid with the soothing effects of glycerin; phenol glycerin, utilizing the antiseptic properties of phenol; and compound iodine paint, also known as Mandl's Paint, which incorporates iodine for its broad-spectrum antimicrobial action. These preparations are typically applied directly to the affected areas using a swab or brush, allowing for targeted treatment of infections and inflammations in the mouth and throat.

Syrups: Syrups are sweet, viscous liquid preparations that play a multifaceted role in pharmaceutical formulations. At their core, syrups are concentrated aqueous solutions of sucrose or other sugars, dissolved in water or another suitable aqueous vehicle. The high sugar concentration serves several purposes beyond merely providing a sweet taste. The Indian Pharmacopoeia (I.P.) defines syrup as a 66.7% w/w solution of sucrose, while the United States Pharmacopeia (U.S.P.) specifies a higher concentration of 85% w/v sucrose in purified water. These high sugar concentrations are not arbitrary; they are carefully chosen to create an environment that is inherently resistant to microbial growth. The high osmotic pressure created by the concentrated sugar solution makes it difficult for most microorganisms to survive, thus acting as a natural preservative.

Syrups with lower sucrose concentrations may require additional preservatives to maintain their stability and prevent microbial contamination. This highlights the delicate balance between sweetness, viscosity, and preservative action in syrup formulations. An interesting phenomenon occurs during the preparation of syrups, particularly when heat is applied. The heating process can cause a slight inversion of sucrose, meaning some sucrose molecules break down into their component monosaccharides, glucose and fructose.

$$\underset{\text{Sucrose}}{C_{12}H_{22}O_{11}} \xrightarrow{H_2O} \underset{\text{Invert sugar}}{2C_6H_{12}O_6}$$

This inversion process can affect the sweetness, viscosity, and stability of the syrup. In some cases, this inversion is desirable as it can prevent crystallization of the sucrose, maintaining the syrup's liquid state.

Syrups serve multiple functions in pharmaceutical preparations:

- As vehicles for active ingredients, especially those with unpleasant tastes.
- As sweetening agents to improve the palatability of medicines, particularly important in pediatric formulations.
- As preservatives, due to their high sugar content.
- As viscosity-enhancing agents, which can aid in the uniform suspension of insoluble particles and slow the settling of dispersed phases.
- Common examples of medicated syrups include cough syrups, where the sweet, viscous nature of the syrup can also provide a soothing effect on the throat, and various vitamin syrups designed for children.

The formulation of syrups requires careful

consideration of factors such as the solubility and stability of active ingredients in high sugar concentrations, potential interactions between ingredients, and the overall stability of the preparation. Proper storage conditions are also crucial to maintain the quality and efficacy of syrup preparations over time.

Elixirs: Elixirs are sophisticated liquid pharmaceutical preparations designed for oral administration. These formulations are characterized by their clarity, pleasant flavor, and sweetened taste, making them particularly palatable to patients. The base of an elixir typically consists of a mixture of ethanol and water, with the alcohol content generally ranging from 15% to 50%. This hydroalcoholic base serves multiple purposes: it acts as a solvent for active ingredients, enhances flavor, and provides some preservative action.

In addition to ethanol and water, elixirs may incorporate other excipients to enhance their properties:

1. Glycerin, sorbitol, or propylene glycol: These agents can improve solubility, enhance sweetness, and contribute to the viscosity of the preparation.
2. Flavoring agents: These are crucial for masking unpleasant tastes of medicinal substances and improving patient compliance.
3. Sugar: While not always present, sugar can enhance sweetness and contribute to the preservation of the elixir.
4. Preservatives: These may be added to prevent microbial growth, especially in elixirs with lower alcohol content.

Elixirs can be categorized into two main types:

1. Medicated elixirs: These contain therapeutic agents, often potent drugs such as antibiotics, antihistamines, or sedatives. The elixir

formulation allows for precise dosing of these potent medications while improving palatability.

2. Non-medicated elixirs: These serve primarily as flavored vehicles for other medications or as pleasant-tasting oral rinses.

Examples of medicated elixirs include Chlorpheniramine elixir (an antihistamine), Diphenhydramine elixir (another antihistamine), and Ephedrine elixir (a decongestant and bronchodilator)

Linctuses: Linctuses are a specific type of oral liquid preparation designed for the treatment of cough. They are characterized by their sweet taste and viscous consistency, which allows them to coat and soothe the throat as they are swallowed. The high viscosity of linctuses is often achieved through the use of sugars, glycerin, or other thickening agents.

Key features of linctuses include:

1. Demulcent properties: Many linctuses contain ingredients that form a soothing film over irritated mucous membranes.
2. Sedative effects: Some linctuses may include ingredients that help suppress the cough reflex.
3. Expectorant properties: Certain linctuses are formulated to help loosen and expel mucus from the respiratory tract.

Linctuses are intended to be swallowed slowly in small doses without the addition of water. This method of administration allows for prolonged contact with the throat tissues, enhancing the therapeutic effect. Examples include Codeine Linctus, which contains the opioid codeine for its cough-suppressant properties, and Noscapine linctus, which uses the non-opioid antitussive noscapine

Nasal Drops: Nasal drops are liquid preparations specifically formulated for administration into the nasal passages. They are typically aqueous solutions, although some may be formulated as emulsions or suspensions. The primary method of application is via a dropper, allowing for precise dosing and targeted delivery to the nasal mucosa.

Nasal drops are commonly used for their:

1. Antiseptic properties: To combat nasal infections
2. Local analgesic effects: To relieve pain or discomfort in the nasal passages
3. Vasoconstrictor action: To reduce nasal congestion by narrowing blood vessels in the nasal tissues

An example of nasal drops is Ephedrine Nasal drops, which utilize the decongestant properties of ephedrine to relieve nasal congestion. The formulation of nasal drops requires careful consideration of factors such as tonicity, pH, and viscosity to ensure comfort and efficacy when applied to the sensitive nasal tissues

Eye drops: Eye drops are specialized pharmaceutical preparations designed for ocular administration. These sterile formulations can be solutions or suspensions and may have an aqueous or oily base, depending on the properties of the active ingredients and the intended therapeutic effect.

Key requirements for eye drop formulations include:

1. Sterility: This is crucial to prevent eye infections.
2. Isotonicity: Eye drops should ideally be isotonic with tear fluid to minimize irritation.
3. Appropriate pH: The pH should be compatible with tear fluid, typically in the range of 7.0-7.4.
4. Buffering: To maintain pH stability and minimize irritation.
5. Absence of foreign particles: To avoid eye

irritation and potential damage.

Eye drops can serve various therapeutic purposes, including:

1. Antiseptic action: To prevent or treat eye infections
2. Anesthetic effects: For local pain relief
3. Anti-inflammatory properties: To reduce ocular inflammation
4. Mydriatic or miotic action: To dilate or constrict the pupil, respectively
5. Diagnostic purposes: Such as fluorescein drops for detecting corneal abrasions

The packaging of eye drops is crucial for maintaining sterility and facilitating easy application. They are typically dispensed in glass or suitable plastic containers with a screw cap fitted with a rubber teat and glass dropper. Alternatively, the container may have a nozzle for direct instillation into the eye.

Examples of eye drops include Atropine eye drops (used for pupil dilation), Chloramphenicol eye drops (an antibiotic for treating eye infections), and Pilocarpine eye drops (used to reduce intraocular pressure in glaucoma patients).

Suspensions: Suspensions are complex biphasic liquid dosage forms that play a significant role in pharmaceutical formulations. They consist of finely divided solid particles, typically ranging from 0.5 to 5 microns in size, suspended or dispersed in a liquid or semi-fluid vehicle. This particle size range is crucial for maintaining stability and ensuring proper therapeutic effect.

Key characteristics of suspensions include:

1. Particle size: The small particle size (0.5-5 microns) ensures a large surface area for drug

dissolution and absorption.

2. Sedimentation rate: Particles in suspension tend to settle over time due to gravity. The rate of sedimentation is influenced by particle size, density difference between particles and medium, and viscosity of the medium.
3. Redispersibility: A well-formulated suspension should be easily redispersed with gentle shaking.
4. Viscosity: The vehicle's viscosity is often adjusted to slow particle settling and improve stability.

Suspensions are utilized for various routes of administration:

1. Oral administration: Common for drugs with poor water solubility or for achieving prolonged drug release.
2. External application: Used in topical preparations for dermatological conditions.
3. Parenteral use: Intramuscular or subcutaneous injections for sustained drug release.

Examples of suspensions include:

- Barium sulphate suspension: Used as a contrast medium in X-ray imaging of the gastrointestinal tract.
- Chalk-Kaolin Suspension: An antacid and adsorbent used for gastrointestinal disturbances.

Formulation challenges in suspensions include maintaining uniformity, preventing caking, and ensuring appropriate rheological properties for the intended use.

Emulsions: Emulsions are sophisticated biphasic liquid dosage forms that enable the mixing of two immiscible liquids through the use of an emulsifying agent (emulgent). This formulation strategy allows for the incorporation of lipophilic drugs into aqueous systems or hydrophilic drugs into lipid systems, enhancing bioavailability and palatability.

Key aspects of emulsions include:

1. Emulsifying agent: This is crucial for stabilizing the emulsion by reducing interfacial tension between the two phases.
2. Droplet size: Typically in the range of 0.1 to 100 micrometers, influencing stability and appearance.
3. Viscosity: Can vary widely depending on the formulation and intended use.

Types of emulsions

1. Oil-in-water (O/W): Oil droplets dispersed in a continuous aqueous phase. These are generally more palatable and used for oral administration.
2. Water-in-oil (W/O): Water droplets dispersed in a continuous oil phase. These are often used for topical applications due to their occlusive properties.

Emulsions offer several advantages:

- Improved palatability compared to taking oils directly
- Enhanced absorption of lipophilic drugs when formulated as O/W emulsions
- Ability to mask unpleasant tastes or odors

Examples of emulsions include:

- Castor oil emulsion: Used as a laxative
- Liquid paraffin emulsion: Used as a moisturizer or mild laxative

It's important to note that emulsions require shaking before use to ensure uniform distribution of the dispersed phase, hence the common label instruction "Shake the bottle before use."

Ointments: Ointments are semi-solid preparations designed for external application to the skin or mucous membranes. They consist of a base in which medicaments are dissolved, suspended, or emulsified. The consistency of ointments allows them to remain in place and provide prolonged contact with the skin, making them ideal for delivering drugs topically.

Key features of ointments include:

1. Occlusive properties: They form a barrier on the skin, reducing water loss and enhancing drug penetration.
2. Emollient action: Many ointment bases have moisturizing properties, benefiting dry or damaged skin.
3. Protective function: They can shield the skin from external irritants or moisture.

Ointment bases can be classified into several categories:

- Hydrocarbon bases (e.g., petrolatum)
- Absorption bases (e.g., lanolin)
- Water-removable bases (e.g., polyethylene glycol ointment)
- Water-soluble bases (e.g., polyethylene glycol)

Examples of ointments include:

- Compound Benzoic Acid ointment: Used as an antifungal preparation
- Cetrimide ointment: An antiseptic preparation

Formulation considerations for ointments include the selection of an appropriate base, ensuring uniform distribution of the active ingredient, and maintaining stability over the product's shelf life

Creams: Creams are semi-solid emulsions that bridge the gap between ointments and lotions in terms of consistency. They are intended for application to the skin and offer several advantages over ointments, including easier application and removal, and a less greasy feel.

Key characteristics of creams include:

1. Lighter consistency compared to ointments
2. Easier to spread and remove
3. Can be either oil-in-water (O/W) or water-in-oil (W/O) emulsions
4. Often preferred by patients due to their cosmetic appeal

Types of creams:

1. O/W creams (vanishing creams): These are absorbed quickly into the skin and are non-greasy.
2. W/O creams: These provide more occlusive effects and are useful for dry skin conditions.

Important considerations for cream formulations:

1. Preservation: Due to their water content, creams are prone to microbial growth. Effective preservatives must be incorporated.
2. Stability: Emulsion stability is crucial to prevent phase separation.
3. pH: Should be compatible with skin pH to avoid irritation.

Examples of creams include Cetomacrogol cream: A base used in various formulations, Chlorhexidine cream: An antiseptic preparation, Hydrocortisone cream: A corticosteroid used for inflammatory skin conditions

Aerosols: Aerosols may be defined as pressurised dosage form of medicament in which the liquid or solid drugs are dissolved or suspended in a gas. The gas used for this purpose is known as propellant. The aerosols are packed in a suitable container known as aerosol container, when pressure is applied to the aerosol system, the contents are expelled out through the opening of the valve in the form of mist, a coarse, wet or dry spray, a stream.

HISTORY OF PHARMACY IN INDIA

In ancient India, medicinal knowledge was derived from plant, animal, and mineral sources. This knowledge was often kept within families and lacked standardized scientific methods. The traditional Indian medical system declined during Muslim rule, while the Unani-Tibbi system gained prominence.

The British colonial period introduced Western or Allopathic medicine to India. Initially reserved for the ruling class, it gradually became popular among the general population by the late 19th century. Before 1940, most drugs were imported from Europe, but domestic production began to emerge with the establishment of facilities like the Bengal Chemical and Pharmaceutical Works in Calcutta (1901) and Alembic Chemical Works in Baroda (1907).

Various legislations were enacted to regulate drugs and related substances. These included the Opium Act (1878), Indian Merchandise Act (1889), and Poisons Act (1919). However, these laws were often insufficient to address the growing pharmaceutical industry's needs.

During World War I, drug imports were disrupted, leading to quality issues and the influx of adulterated or inferior medicines. This situation highlighted the need for more comprehensive regulations.

In response to these challenges, the Indian government appointed the Drug Enquiry Committee in 1930, chaired by Col. R.N. Chopra. The committee's report, published in 1931, revealed the lack of a specialized pharmacy profession in India.

Significant developments in pharmaceutical

education and professional organizations followed. Prof. M.L. Schroff initiated university-level pharmaceutical education at Banaras Hindu University. The Indian Pharmaceutical Association was established in 1935, and the Indian Journal of Pharmacy was launched in 1939.

Key legislative milestones included:

- The Drugs Act of 1940, regulating drug import, manufacture, sale, and distribution
- The Pharmacy Act of 1948, standardizing pharmacy education
- The publication of the Indian Pharmacopoeial List in 1946
- The establishment of the Pharmacy Council of India in 1949
- The Drugs and Magic Remedies (Objectionable Advertisements) Act of 1954
- The Narcotic and Psychotropic Substances Act of 1985

HISTORY OF PHARMACY EDUCATION

The evolution of pharmacy education in India can be traced to the first pharmacy course started in December 1860 at the Madras Medical College. At that time, students were taught the art of compounding, dispensing and labeling the instructions for use of various pharmacopoeial preparations. Later, a certified two year diploma course for Chemists and Druggists was stared at Madras Medical College and in Visakhapatnam in 1937. Sudents who had attended the courses in Materia medica, chemistry and practical pharmacy were awarded the certificate of Chemists and Druggists. Compounder courses were also started in Bengal, Bihar, Bombay and

Uttar Pradesh. An advanced sustem of pharmaceutical education comprising a diploma course in pharmacy was being taught at the school of pharmacy, Panaji, in Goa which was a Portugese colony.

The Modern Pharmacy Education

The modern pharmacy education evolved with the established of the first degree level course in pharmacy in Banaras Hindu University (BHU) IN 1932. Professor Mahadev Lal Schroff is regarded as father of modern pharmacy for this pivotal role in starting a two year bachelor course course in pharmaceutical chemistry (B.Sc Pharmaceutical Chemistry). In July 1937, a three year degree course, Bachelor of Pharmacy (B.Pharm) was started in he Department of pharmaceutics of BHU under the services of prominent teachers like G.P Srivatsava, N.K. Basu, G.B. Singh, S. Prasad, D.N. Majumdar and N.C. Neogi. The interest in pharmaceutical education and various universities across the country like Andhra University, Madras Medical College (University of Madras), Department of Chemical Technology(University of Bombay), Punjab University and Lallubhai Motilal college of Pharmacy, Ahmedabad started degree level pharmacy course.

In 1950, Prof. M.L. Schroff started the Department of pharmacy at the Birla College (Presently BITS, Pilani). The university of Sangar (now Dr. Hari Singh Gaur Viswavidyalaya) and university of Nagpur were the other prominent institutions who started B. Pharm courses at that time. As the B. Pharm degree level education flourished far and wide, post-graduate education in pharmacy was also pioneered on parallel grounds. In April 1940, Banaras Hindu University introduced a one year course of research that awarded the degree of Master of Pharmacy. Between 1952-53, the duration of M.Pharm course was increased to 1.5 years and the curriculum compromised classroom instruction in recent advancements in pharmacy and chemistry of drugs. The other universities that introduced M. Pharm were Punjab University, Andhra University, University of Sangar, University of Madras, Birla College, Pilani and Department of Pharmacology, SMS Medical college, Jaipur. In the later years, programmes of research leading to Doctor Philosophy (Ph. D), degree in pharmacy were started. In September 1994, the Government, made a very significant development in pharmaceutical education with the establishment of National Institute of Pharmaceutical Education and Research at Mohali, Punjab under the directorship of Dr. C.L. Kaul. B.V. Patel Pharmaceutical Education and Research Development Centre established in September 1990 near Ahmedabad under the directorship of H.L. Bhalla.

HISTORY OF THE PROFESSION OF PHARMACY IN INDIA IN RELATION TO INDUSTRY

PRE-INDEPENDENCE ERA

1. For the First time in India, a chemist shop was opened in 1811 in Calcutta by Mr. Bathgate who came to India through East India Company. In 1910, this form started manufacture of Tinctures and spirits.

2. Another firm, Smith Stanistree and Co., started Apothecary shop in 1821 and commenced the manufacturing in 1918.

3. Bengal Chemicals and Pharmaceutical Works, a small factory was started in Calcutta in 1901, by Acharya Prafulla Chandra Roy

4. In 1903, under the leadership of Prof. T.K. Gajjar, a

small factory at Parel was started which led to the development of other pharmaceutical units, like Alembic Chemical Works Ltd., at Baroda.

5. The other relatively big units added during the early part of the centuary were the Sarabhai Chemical works, Bengal Immunity Laboratory and a few governmental laboratories for the manufacture of vaccines and sera.

6. Modern Drug Research in India started in 1920, when Sir Ramnath Chopra setup an active research centre at the school of Tropical medicine in Calcutta.

7. The efforts of Dr. Upendranath Brahmachari at the Camp-bell Medical School, Calcutta led to the introduction of Urea Stibamine in 1922 for the treatment of Kala-Azar.

8. During World war-I, when the local demand of allopathic medicines increased sharply and imports got completely cut off, a number of foreign and National residents who had experience in Ayurvedic preparations started manufacturing simple cough syrups, tablets and capsules.

9. Production of Quinine salts was taken up in government factories in Darjeeling and Nilgiris which had been up earlier.

10. By 1930, the manufacturing of biological like Sera and vaccines, Anaesthetics like Ether, Chloroform, few simple drugs like based on coal tar distillation products began in The country.

11. With the outbreak of World war-II, Indian Pharmaceutical Indutry started undertaking the production of no. of plant based, synthetic and biological

12. It was during this period, the manufacture of Anti-dysentry drugs like Iodochlor, Chemotherapeutic drugs like Arsenical, Antileprotic drugs and colloidal preparations of Calcium, Silver, Iodine etc was started. Also the production of biological like liver extracts,

pituitary extracts and Adrenaline solution was taken up

13. To co-ordinate the various activities of Industrial Research and Development in India, CSIR was registered on Mar 12, 1942

14. However, till Independence, pharmaceutical Industry remained relatively small and the production was confined mainly to galenicals, simple formulations, some vaccines and sera. The total production when India became independent was around 10 crore.

POST INDEPENDENCE ERA

1. Realising the role of pharmaceutical Industry, the Govt. of India paid a special attention to the needs of this industry. In 1948, a survey was carried out and a programme of development was undertaken in the first five years which was subsequently followed every five years.

2. Inorder to reduce the dependency on import and to increase the production of Antibiotics, "Hindusthan Antibiotics Ltd.," was set up in 1954 at Pimpri near Pune.

3. In the early 1960's the Indigenisation of the Industry started R&D collaboration between the Industries, National laboratories and academia. The Indian Drugs and Pharmaceutical Ltd., was set up by the Government n 1964 to provide a boost to the production of bulk drugs and formulations.

4. The 1970's saw an upsurge of R&D within the Industry the Industry because of the encouragement provided by the Government to establish R&D units within the Industry in the form of liberal tariff, tax concessions and financial incentives

5. Special provision in Patent Act 1970, to exclude product patents for drugs and medicines, food and chemical provided the right climate for technology innovation.

6. The 1980's and 1990's saw the setting up of drug manufacturing units both in the organized and unorganised sectors

PRESENT STATUS

Presently, Indian Pharmaceutical Industry is estimated to a $10 billion industry with drastic Industry expansion in the last two decades. Pharmaceutical Industry in India is highly competitive sector with more than 23,000 registered units of which 300 are large scale companies and 10,000 small companies including 5 central public sector units. Leading 300 pharmaceutical companies contribute to 70% of the total Indian pharmaceutical industry produces 70,000 different drugs and the most important segment of domestic market is the anti-infectives accounting for one-quarter of total turnover followed by cardiovascular preparations, cold remedies and pain killers each accounting for one-tenth f the total turnover.

Some of the India's major pharma companies like Nicholas Piramal, Wockhardt, Sun Pharma, Cipla, Aurabindo, Ranbaxy, Dr. Reddy's have achieved world class technological infrastructure during the past few years. India ranks 14th in terms of value and 3rd in terms of volume of drugs produced, as Indian economic survey report 2009-2010. Statistics revealed that Indian pharma Industry has grown from 1500 crore turnover in 1980 to 78,000 crores in 2008. It registered 14% growth rate in bulk drugs and 20% growth rate in formulations during 2007-2008. Indian Pharma Industry has grown consistently at 9.5% CAGR compared to 7% annual growth rate of the world market.

HISTORY OF THE PROFESSION OF PHARMACY PRACTICE IN INDIA

The history of the pharmacy practice in India is a fascinating journey that spans centuries and reflects the evolution of healthcare practices, trade routes, and cultural influences. The practice of pharmacy in India has deep roots, dating back to ancient times when traditional systems of medicine, such as Ayurveda, Siddha, and Unani, were flourishing.

1. **Ancient Period:** The earliest mentions of pharmaceutical practices in India can be traced back to the Vedas, the ancient Indian scriptures. Ayurveda, the traditional system of medicine, provided a comprehensive understanding of medicinal plants, their properties, and methods of preparation. The Charaka Samhita and Sushruta Samhita, ancient Ayurvedic texts, documented pharmaceutical knowledge and practices.
2. **Islamic Influence:** With the advent of Islamic rule in the Indian subcontinent, the Unani system of medicine gained prominence. Unani, with its roots in Greek medicine, was further developed by Islamic scholars. This period saw the establishment of pharmacies attached to hospitals and the standardization of drug formulations.
3. **Colonial Era:** The colonial period significantly influenced the practice of pharmacy in India. The British East India Company introduced Western medical practices, and with it, the concept of modern pharmacy. Western pharmaceutical education began with the establishment of the Calcutta School of Pharmacy in 1823. The profession saw further developments with the establishment of the Indian Pharmaceutical Congress in 1948.
4. **Post-Independence Era:** After gaining independence in 1947, India witnessed significant advancements in pharmaceutical education, research, and industry.

The Pharmacy Act of 1948 was a landmark legislation that regulated the profession and established the Pharmacy Council of India. The establishment of pharmacy colleges and universities further contributed to the growth of the profession.

5. **Globalization and Industry Growth:** In the late 20th century and early 21st century, India's pharmaceutical industry gained global recognition. The country became a major player in the production of generic drugs, and Indian pharmacists contributed to research and development in the pharmaceutical sector on a global scale.
6. **Regulatory Changes:** The regulatory landscape of pharmacy practice in India has evolved over the years. The Drugs and Cosmetics Act of 1940 and subsequent amendments have played a crucial role in regulating the manufacture, sale, and distribution of drugs. The National Pharmaceutical Pricing Authority (NPPA) was established to regulate drug prices and ensure affordability.
7. **Challenges and Opportunities:** The pharmacy profession in India faces challenges such as counterfeit drugs, inadequate regulatory enforcement, and the need for continuous professional development. However, opportunities for pharmacists have expanded with the growing healthcare industry, pharmaceutical research, and advancements in technology.
8. **Current Scenario:** In the present day, the pharmacy profession in India is diverse, encompassing community pharmacy, hospital pharmacy, industrial pharmacy, and regulatory affairs. The role of pharmacists extends beyond dispensing medications to active involvement in patient care, drug information services, and public health initiatives.

HISTORY OF VARIOUS PHARMACY PROFESSIONAL ASSOCIATIONS

The history of pharmacy professional associations in India is integral to the growth and development of the pharmacy profession in the country. These associations have played a crucial role in bringing together pharmacists, promoting education and research, and advocating for the interests of the pharmacy community. Several notable pharmacy organizations have made significant contributions to shaping the landscape of pharmaceutical practice in India.

1. **Indian Pharmaceutical Association (IPA):** Founded in 1939, the Indian Pharmaceutical Association (IPA) is one of the oldest and most prominent pharmacy associations in India. It has been instrumental in promoting the pharmaceutical profession, fostering research, and providing a platform for pharmacists to exchange knowledge. The IPA has been actively involved in advocating for the interests of pharmacists and contributing to policy discussions related to the pharmaceutical industry.
2. **Pharmacy Council of India (PCI):** The Pharmacy Council of India (PCI) was established in 1948 under the Pharmacy Act. It serves as the regulatory body for the pharmacy profession in India. The PCI is responsible for setting and maintaining educational standards for pharmacy courses, registering pharmacists, and regulating pharmacy practice. It plays a pivotal role in ensuring the quality of pharmacy education and safeguarding the professional interests of pharmacists.
3. **Indian Hospital Pharmacists Association (IHPA):** The Indian Hospital Pharmacists Association (IHPA)

was founded in 1980 to address the specific needs and challenges faced by hospital pharmacists. This association focuses on promoting the role of pharmacists in hospital settings, enhancing patient care through rational drug use, and providing a platform for hospital pharmacists to share their experiences and expertise.

4. **Association of Pharmaceutical Teachers of India (APTI):** Formed in 1966, the Association of Pharmaceutical Teachers of India (APTI) is dedicated to the professional development of pharmacy educators. APTI aims to enhance the quality of pharmacy education, facilitate research in pharmaceutical sciences, and provide a forum for educators to collaborate and share best practices. It has played a vital role in shaping the academic landscape of pharmacy in India.
5. **All India Drugs Control Officers' Confederation (AIDCOC):** The All India Drugs Control Officers' Confederation (AIDCOC) represents the drug control officers across the country. Established to address issues related to drug regulation and control, AIDCOC works towards promoting effective drug administration and ensuring the safety and efficacy of pharmaceuticals.
6. **Indian Pharmacological Society (IPS):** The Indian Pharmacological Society (IPS) was founded in 1969 and is dedicated to the advancement of pharmacology and related sciences. While not exclusively a pharmacy association, IPS plays a crucial role in promoting research and education in pharmacology, which has significant implications for the pharmaceutical field.

These associations, among others, have been essential in fostering a sense of community among pharmacists, addressing professional challenges, and contributing to the growth and recognition of the pharmacy profession in India. Through their various activities, these organizations continue to shape the future of pharmacy by promoting excellence in education, research, and practice

Pharmacy as a career

Pharmacy as a career offers a diverse and rewarding path for individuals interested in healthcare, science, and patient well-being. Pharmacists, as healthcare professionals, play a crucial role in the safe and effective use of medications, ensuring patient health and contributing to the broader healthcare system. Here's an exploration of pharmacy as a career, covering education, roles, responsibilities, and opportunities:

1. **Educational Path:** The journey to becoming a pharmacist typically involves a formal education in pharmacy. In many countries, including the United States and India, aspiring pharmacists pursue a Bachelor of Pharmacy (B.Pharm) or Doctor of Pharmacy (Pharm.D) degree. The latter is a postgraduate program that provides a more comprehensive education and often includes clinical rotations. In some regions, additional licensing or certification exams may be required.
2. **Roles and Responsibilities:** Pharmacists play diverse roles in different settings, including:
    - **Community Pharmacy:** Interacting directly with patients, dispensing medications, providing advice on over-the-counter drugs, and offering health and wellness information.
    - **Hospital Pharmacy:** Collaborating with healthcare teams to ensure proper medication use within a hospital setting, including

managing drug distribution and monitoring patient outcomes.

- **Clinical Pharmacy:** Working closely with healthcare providers to optimize medication therapy, manage chronic conditions, and ensure patient safety.
- **Industrial Pharmacy:** Involvement in drug manufacturing, quality control, and research and development within pharmaceutical companies.

3. **Patient-Centric Focus:** One of the distinguishing features of a pharmacy career is its strong patient-centric focus. Pharmacists often serve as accessible healthcare professionals, answering questions, providing counseling on medications, and promoting medication adherence. This direct patient interaction contributes significantly to overall patient care.
4. **Professional Development:** The field of pharmacy encourages continuous learning and professional development. Pharmacists stay updated on the latest drug therapies, advancements in pharmaceutical sciences, and changes in healthcare regulations. Continuing education and participation in professional organizations help pharmacists enhance their skills and stay at the forefront of their field.
5. **Job Outlook and Opportunities:** The demand for pharmacists remains robust globally. In addition to traditional roles in community and hospital pharmacies, pharmacists are increasingly sought after in roles such as pharmaceutical research, regulatory affairs, academia, and healthcare administration. The evolving landscape of healthcare, pharmaceuticals, and biotechnology opens up new and exciting career paths for pharmacists.
6. **Global Impact:** Pharmacy is a globally recognized

profession, and pharmacists contribute significantly to public health. Their involvement in drug development, distribution, and counseling has a direct impact on the well-being of individuals and communities. The profession's global nature also allows for opportunities to work in different countries and contribute to international health initiatives.

7. **Technological Integration:** The pharmacy profession has embraced technological advancements. Pharmacists use sophisticated pharmacy management systems, digital health tools, and telepharmacy services to enhance patient care and streamline medication-related processes

Summary

The profession of pharmacy has undergone a remarkable transformation over millennia, evolving from ancient healing practices to a sophisticated scientific discipline. Early civilizations in Mesopotamia, Egypt, and China laid the foundation with herbal remedies and primitive medicinal preparations, documented in early texts like the Ebers Papyrus. Greek and Roman influences, particularly through figures like Hippocrates and Galen, shaped the theoretical framework of pharmacy, introducing concepts of humoral theory and systematic approaches to medicine. The Middle Ages saw monasteries become bastions of medical knowledge, with monks meticulously copying and preserving ancient texts while developing new remedies. As Europe emerged from this period, apothecaries rose to prominence, marking the beginnings of pharmacy as a distinct profession. The Renaissance ushered in advancements in botanical studies and chemical processes, setting the stage for modern pharmacology. The Industrial Revolution brought about a paradigm shift with the rise of pharmaceutical manufacturing, gradually separating pharmacy from medicine. The 20th century witnessed unprecedented progress, from the discovery of antibiotics to the development of sophisticated synthetic drugs, revolutionizing healthcare. Pharmacy education evolved from apprenticeship models to rigorous university programs, reflecting the increasing complexity of the field. The profession's scope expanded to include clinical roles, emphasizing patient care and medication management. Specializations like nuclear pharmacy and pharmacoepidemiology emerged, broadening the field's impact. Today, pharmacy stands at the forefront of healthcare innovation, embracing personalized medicine, biotechnology, and digital health solutions, while pharmacists play pivotal roles in interdisciplinary healthcare teams, shaping the future of global health.

Multiple Choice Questions

1. Which ancient civilization is credited with the first known pharmaceutical text, the Ebers Papyrus?
   a) Greek
   b) Roman
   c) Egyptian
   d) Chinese
2. Who is considered the "Father of Pharmacy"?
   a) Hippocrates
   b) Galen
   c) Avicenna
   d) Paracelsus
3. In which century did pharmacy and medicine begin to separate as distinct professions?

a) 11th century
b) 13th century
c) 15th century
d) 17th century

4. The first official pharmacopoeia was published in:
   a) England
   b) France
   c) Germany
   d) Italy
5. Which of the following was NOT a major contribution of Arabic pharmacy to the field?
   a) Development of syrups and juleps
   b) Introduction of distillation techniques
   c) Creation of the first synthetic drug
   d) Establishment of the first apothecary shops
6. The term "pharmacy" is derived from the Greek word "pharmakon," which means:
   a) Medicine
   b) Poison
   c) Both medicine and poison
   d) Healing
7. Which event significantly impacted the development of pharmacy in the 20th century?
   a) The Industrial Revolution
   b) World War II
   c) The discovery of penicillin
   d) The invention of the computer
8. The first college of pharmacy in the United States was established in:
   a) New York
   b) Philadelphia
   c) Boston
   d) Chicago
9. Which of the following is considered a milestone in the history of pharmacy education?

a) Introduction of the PharmD program
b) Establishment of the first pharmacy school
c) Development of the first synthetic drug
d) Creation of the first pharmacopoeia

10. The concept of "pharmaceutical care" was introduced in:
a) 1960s
b) 1970s
c) 1980s
d) 1990s

11. Which ancient Greek physician is known for his work "De Materia Medica," an early precursor to modern pharmacopoeias?
a) Hippocrates
b) Galen
c) Dioscorides
d) Aristotle

12. The first woman to receive a degree in pharmacy in the United States was:
a) Elizabeth Blackwell
b) Mary Corinna Putnam Jacobi
c) Susan Hayhurst
d) Margaret Rudkin

13. Which of the following contributed to the standardization of drug manufacturing in the early 20th century?
a) The Pure Food and Drug Act of 1906
b) The discovery of insulin
c) The invention of the tablet press
d) The establishment of the World Health Organization

14. The practice of compounding medications:
a) Began in the 20th century
b) Was phased out completely with industrialization

c) Continues to be an important aspect of pharmacy practice
d) Is only practiced in developing countries

15. Which of the following is NOT a major area of modern pharmacy practice?
a) Community pharmacy
b) Hospital pharmacy
c) Industrial pharmacy
d) Astrological pharmacy

16. The development of clinical pharmacy as a discipline began in:
a) 1940s
b) 1950s
c) 1960s
d) 1970s

17. Which technological advancement has significantly impacted pharmacy practice in recent decades?
a) Electronic health records
b) Automated dispensing systems
c) Online pharmacies
d) All of the above

18. The concept of "pharmaceutical equivalence" is important in:
a) Drug discovery
b) Generic drug development
c) Pharmacoeconomics
d) Pharmacovigilance

19. Which of the following best describes the role of a modern pharmacist?
a) Solely dispensing medications
b) Manufacturing drugs
c) Providing patient-centered care and medication management
d) Conducting clinical trials

20. The shift towards patient-centered care in pharmacy practice is known as:
    a) Clinical pharmacy
    b) Pharmaceutical care
    c) Community pharmacy
    d) Hospital pharmacy

List of Important Questions

1. What were the major contributions of ancient civilizations (e.g., Egyptian, Greek, Roman) to the development of pharmacy?
2. How did Islamic pharmacy influence the development of the profession in Europe during the Middle Ages?
3. What role did alchemists play in the evolution of pharmacy and medicinal chemistry?
4. Who was Galen, and how did his work impact pharmaceutical practice?
5. Describe the significance of Paracelsus in the history of pharmacy and medicine.
6. How did the establishment of apothecary shops in medieval Europe contribute to the profession's development?
7. What was the impact of the Industrial Revolution on pharmaceutical manufacturing and practice?
8. Discuss the evolution of pharmaceutical education from apprenticeship to formal academic programs.
9. How did the discovery of penicillin by Alexander Fleming revolutionize pharmacy and medicine?
10. What were the key milestones in the development of modern pharmaceutical regulations?
11. How has the role of pharmacists evolved from compounders to medication therapy managers?
12. Discuss the impact of computerization and automation on pharmacy practice.
13. What are the major differences between traditional pharmacy practice and clinical pharmacy?
14. How has the concept of pharmaceutical care transformed the profession of pharmacy?
15. What are the current trends and future prospects in the field of pharmacy?

Bibliography

1. Sonnedecker G. Kremers and Urdang's History of pharmacy. 4th ed. Madison: American Institute of the History of Pharmacy; 1986.
2. Anderson S. Making medicines: a brief history of pharmacy and pharmaceuticals. London: Pharmaceutical Press; 2005.
3. Higby GJ. From compounding to caring: an abridged history of American pharmacy. In: Knowlton CH, Penna RP, editors. Pharmaceutical care. New York: Chapman and Hall; 1996. p. 18-45.
4. Buerki RA, Vottero LD. Pharmacy ethics: a foundation for professional practice. Washington, DC: American Pharmacists Association; 2013.
5. Hepler CD, Strand LM. Opportunities and responsibilities in pharmaceutical care. Am J Hosp Pharm. 1990;47(3):533-43.
6. Brock WH. Justus von Liebig: the chemical gatekeeper. Cambridge: Cambridge University Press; 1997.
7. Hadzović S. Pharmacy and the great contribution of Arab-Islamic science to its development. Med Arh. 1997;51(1-2):47-50.
8. Cowen DL, Helfand WH. Pharmacy: an illustrated history. New York: Harry N. Abrams; 1990.
9. Mrtek RG, Catizone C. Pharmacy and the professions. In: Gennaro AR, editor. Remington: The science and practice of pharmacy. 20th ed. Philadelphia: Lippincott Williams & Wilkins; 2000. p. 1-19.
10. Buerki RA. In search of excellence: the first century of the American Association of Colleges of Pharmacy. Alexandria: American Association of Colleges of Pharmacy; 1999.

CHAPTER 2

PHARMACOPOEIAS

Author

Dr Vijaykumar Darshanam,
HOD and Professor, Department of Pharmaceutics, Swami Vivekananda Institute of Pharmaceutical Sciences, Yadagirigutta, Yadadri Bhongir, Telangana, India

Abstract

Pharmacopoeias serve as authoritative compendia of standards for pharmaceutical substances, playing a crucial role in ensuring drug quality, safety, and efficacy. These official publications provide detailed specifications for the identity, purity, and quality of drugs and excipients. The concept of pharmacopoeias dates back to ancient medical texts, evolving into standardized references for modern pharmaceutical practice. Today, major pharmacopoeias such as the United States Pharmacopeia, British Pharmacopoeia, and European Pharmacopoeia are regularly updated to reflect advances in pharmaceutical science and technology. These compendia contain monographs detailing drug descriptions, identification tests, purity criteria, assay methods, and storage requirements. Pharmacopoeias also include general chapters on analytical methods, dosage form standards, and quality control procedures. The development and revision of pharmacopoeial standards involve collaborative efforts between regulatory bodies, industry experts, and academic researchers. Efforts towards international harmonization aim to streamline global pharmaceutical trade and ensure consistent drug quality worldwide. Understanding and applying pharmacopoeial standards is essential for pharmaceutical professionals in drug development, manufacturing, and quality assurance

Keywords: *Monograph, Drug standards, Quality control, Regulatory compliance, Harmonization, Pharmaceutical analysis*

Learning Objectives

After completion of the chapter, the student should be able to:

- Define pharmacopoeia and explain its importance in pharmaceutical practice.
- Compare and contrast different national and international pharmacopoeias.
- Describe the structure and organization of a typical pharmacopoeia.
- Explain the process of creating and updating pharmacopoeial monographs.
- Identify the key information provided in pharmacopoeial monographs.
- Discuss the role of pharmacopoeias in ensuring drug quality and standardization.
- Analyze the legal and regulatory aspects of pharmacopoeias in different countries.

The drug compendia, including pharmacopoeias and formularies, are essential resources in the pharmaceutical industry. They contain standardized information about drugs and related substances, including their sources, descriptions, standards, tests, preparation methods, actions, uses, dosages, and storage conditions.

These compendia are typically prepared under government authority and are regularly revised to incorporate the latest information. They serve as legal standards for drug purity, quality, and strength in their respective countries.

Drug compendia are classified into two main categories:

1. Official Compendia:
   These are legally recognized standards in their

countries of origin. Examples include:

- British Pharmacopoeia (BP)
- Indian Pharmacopoeia (IP)
- United States Pharmacopoeia (USP)
- National Formulary (NF)

2. Non-Official Compendia: These serve as secondary reference sources and include:

- Merck Index
- Extra Pharmacopoeia (Martindale)
- United States Dispensatory

The Indian Pharmacopoeia (IP) has a rich history dating back to 1563. Key milestones include:

- 1841: Bengal Pharmacopoeia and Conspectus of Drugs
- 1946: Indian Pharmacopoeial List
- 1955: First edition of Indian Pharmacopoeia
- 1966: Second edition
- 1985: Third edition
- 1996: Fourth edition

The IP is prepared with input from pharmaceutical industry experts, drug control laboratories, and research institutions. It serves as the official standard for drugs and related substances in India under the Drugs and Cosmetics Act 1940.

The development of the IP reflects India's growing pharmaceutical industry and the need for standardized, locally relevant drug information. Its regular updates ensure that it remains a vital resource for maintaining drug quality and safety in the country

VARIOUS OFFICIAL PUBLICATIONS RELATED TO PHARMACY PROFESSION IN INDIA

1. NATIONAL FORMULARY OF INDIA

The National Formulary of India serves as an essential guide for medical practitioners, students, and pharmacists in hospitals and sales departments. First published in 1960 by the Government of India's Ministry of Health, it has seen subsequent editions in 1966 and 1979. This comprehensive resource offers valuable information on various aspects of drug use, including drug interactions, resistance, cumulative effects, and drug dependence. It also provides guidance on proper prescription writing techniques. The National Formulary of India plays a crucial role in standardizing pharmaceutical practices across the country and ensuring that healthcare professionals have access to up-to-date, reliable information on medications and their proper use.

2. THE INDIAN PHARMACOPOEIA

The Indian Pharmacopoeia holds official status under the Drugs and Cosmetics Act 1940, serving as the authoritative source for drug standards in India. Its journey began with the publication of the Indian Pharmacopoeial List in 1946, followed by the first edition of the Indian Pharmacopoeia in 1955. Over the years, it has undergone several revisions and updates, with new editions and supplements published regularly to keep pace with advancements in pharmaceutical science. The fourth edition, published in 1996, represents the culmination of decades of work in standardizing drug information for the Indian market. Each monograph in the Indian Pharmacopoeia provides detailed information on chemical structures, molecular weights, physical descriptions, solubility, identification tests, standards, assay methods, and storage requirements for individual drugs. This comprehensive approach ensures that pharmaceutical manufacturers in India adhere to stringent quality standards, promoting the safety and efficacy of medications available in the country

3. THE BRITISH PHARMACOPOEIA (BP)

The British Pharmacopoeia, first published in 1864, has a rich history spanning over 150 years. Initially authorized under the Medical Act 1858, its responsibility was later transferred to the Medicines Commission in 1968 under the Medicines Act. The BP has undergone numerous revisions and updates, with significant editions published in 1932, 1980, 1988, and 1993. The 1988 edition, for example, comprised two volumes containing over 2,100 monographs. Volume I focused on medicinal and pharmaceutical substances, including infrared reference spectra, while Volume II covered formulated preparations, blood products, immunological products, radiopharmaceutical preparations, surgical materials, and appendices. As a cornerstone of pharmaceutical standards in the United Kingdom and many Commonwealth countries, the British Pharmacopoeia continues to play a vital role in ensuring the quality and consistency of medications across these regions.

4. BRITISH PHARMACEUTICAL CODEX (BPC)

The British Pharmaceutical Codex, initiated in 1903 and first published in 1907, was developed by the Pharmaceutical Society of Great Britain as a reference book for medical practitioners and dispensing pharmacists. In 1959, at the request of the British Pharmacopoeia Commission, the publication of the Codex was synchronized with that of the BP to ensure consistency in the implementation of pharmaceutical standards. The BPC differs from the BP in several key aspects. It includes a broader range of drugs and preparations, some of which may be included in advance of their inclusion in the pharmacopoeia, while others may have been retained from former editions due to their continued common use. Additionally, the BPC provides more comprehensive information on drug actions, uses, undesirable effects, precautions, and toxicology. It also includes formulae, preparation methods, and storage conditions for extemporaneously prepared pharmacy items, making it an invaluable resource for pharmacists engaged in compounding

5. THE UNITED STATES PHARMACOPOEIA (USP)

The United States Pharmacopoeia, first published in 1820, has a long-standing history as the authoritative source for drug standards in the United States. It was originally published under the authority of the United States Pharmacopoeial Convention. In parallel, the National Formulary (NF) was established in 1888 by the American Pharmaceutical Association. A significant development occurred in 1974 when the USP Convention acquired the NF. This acquisition led to the merger of these two important resources, resulting in the publication of a single, comprehensive official book of drug standards known as The United States Pharmacopoeia and The National Formulary (USP-NF) from 1980 onwards. This consolidation has streamlined the process of maintaining and updating drug standards in the United States, providing a unified reference for pharmaceutical quality and consistency.

6. EXTRA PHARMACOPOEIA

The Extra Pharmacopoeia, commonly known as "Martindale," was first produced in 1883 by William Martindale. This authoritative reference book on drugs has gained worldwide recognition and use. Published under the direction of the Council of the Royal Pharmaceutical Society of Great Britain and prepared in the Society's Department of Pharmaceutical Sciences, the Extra Pharmacopoeia provides comprehensive and up-to-date information on drugs and medicines. Its scope extends beyond official pharmacopoeias, offering a wealth of additional data on pharmaceutical substances, their properties, uses, and interactions. The continuous updates and revisions of Martindale ensure that it remains a vital resource for healthcare professionals, providing them with the latest information necessary for safe and effective drug therapy.

7. NATIONAL FORMULARY (NF)

A National Formulary (NF) is a comprehensive and authoritative compilation of drug standards and specifications that serves as a reference guide for healthcare professionals, pharmacists, and regulatory authorities. The primary purpose of a National Formulary is to establish and maintain standards for the identity, quality, purity, strength, and consistency of drugs and their dosage forms.

Key aspects of a National Formulary include:

1. **Standardization of Medications:** National Formularies provide a standardized reference for the composition and characteristics of pharmaceutical products. They establish criteria for the quality and purity of drugs to ensure

consistency in manufacturing and use.

2. **Inclusion of Monographs:** Monographs within a National Formulary provide detailed information about individual drugs, including their chemical structure, pharmacological properties, dosage forms, recommended dosages, contraindications, and other relevant information. These monographs serve as a comprehensive resource for healthcare professionals to make informed decisions about drug therapy.
3. **Regulatory Compliance:** National Formularies often serve as regulatory tools, helping regulatory authorities set and enforce standards for drug manufacturing, distribution, and dispensing. Compliance with the specifications outlined in the National Formulary is essential for ensuring the safety and efficacy of pharmaceutical products.
4. **Promotion of Interchangeability:** National Formularies may provide guidelines for the interchangeability of generic and brand-name drugs. This promotes cost-effectiveness in healthcare by allowing pharmacists to substitute equivalent medications without compromising therapeutic efficacy or safety.
5. **Updates and Revisions:** A National Formulary is a dynamic document that requires regular updates to reflect advances in pharmaceutical science, changes in therapeutic guidelines, and the introduction of new medications. These updates ensure that the information remains current and relevant.
6. **International Collaboration:** While the term "National Formulary" implies a focus on a specific country, many nations collaborate with

international organizations to harmonize drug standards globally. This collaboration is crucial for ensuring the consistency of pharmaceutical products across borders, especially as the pharmaceutical industry becomes increasingly globalized.

7. **Pharmacopeias and Compendia:** National Formularies are often associated with pharmacopeias and compendia, which are additional references that provide standards for drugs, drug substances, and pharmaceutical ingredients. Examples include the United States Pharmacopeia (USP), the British Pharmacopoeia (BP), and the European Pharmacopoeia (Ph. Eur.).
8. **Educational Resource:** National Formularies serve as valuable educational resources for pharmacy students, healthcare practitioners, and researchers. They contribute to the dissemination of knowledge about drug formulations, dosages, and standards.

Examples of National Formularies include the United States Pharmacopeia-National Formulary (USP-NF), the Indian Pharmacopoeia (IP), and the British National Formulary (BNF). Each of these plays a crucial role in ensuring the quality and safety of pharmaceutical products within their respective regions.

Summary

Pharmacopoeias stand as cornerstones of pharmaceutical standardization, evolving from ancient herbals to comprehensive compendia of drug standards essential for ensuring medicinal quality, safety, and efficacy. These authoritative texts trace their origins to early dispensatories in Renaissance Europe, with the first official pharmacopoeia published in Florence in 1498. Major pharmacopoeias like the British Pharmacopoeia, United States Pharmacopeia, and European Pharmacopoeia have developed over centuries, continuously adapting to advances in pharmaceutical science and technology. Modern pharmacopoeias are structured with meticulous detail, featuring monographs that provide specifications for active ingredients, excipients, and finished dosage forms. These standards are established through rigorous scientific processes involving expert committees and public consultations, ensuring they reflect the latest knowledge and best practices in pharmaceutical manufacturing and analysis. Analytical methods described in pharmacopoeias encompass a wide range of techniques, from classical wet chemistry to sophisticated instrumental analyses like high-performance liquid chromatography and mass spectrometry. The concept of pharmacopoeial reference standards plays a crucial role in quality control, providing benchmarks for the industry. Pharmacopoeias hold legal status in many countries, forming an integral part of regulatory frameworks governing drug production and distribution. The challenges of keeping pace with rapidly advancing pharmaceutical technologies and emerging therapies, such as biotechnology products and personalized medicines, drive continuous revision and expansion of these compendia. International harmonization efforts, spearheaded by initiatives like the Pharmacopoeial Discussion Group and the International Conference on Harmonisation, aim to align standards globally, facilitating international trade and ensuring consistent drug quality worldwide.

Multiple Choice Questions

1. What is the primary purpose of a pharmacopoeia?
   a) To list all available medications
   b) To provide standards for drug quality and purity
   c) To give dosing instructions for medications
   d) To regulate drug pricing
2. Which of the following is considered the oldest continuously published pharmacopoeia?
   a) British Pharmacopoeia
   b) United States Pharmacopeia
   c) European Pharmacopoeia
   d) Japanese Pharmacopoeia
3. The International Pharmacopoeia is published by:
   a) World Health Organization (WHO)
   b) International Pharmaceutical Federation (FIP)
   c) United Nations (UN)
   d) World Trade Organization (WTO)
4. Which pharmacopoeia is used as the official standard in the United States?
   a) British Pharmacopoeia
   b) United States Pharmacopeia
   c) European Pharmacopoeia
   d) International Pharmacopoeia
5. The monographs in a pharmacopoeia typically include information on:
   a) Chemical structure of drugs

b) Methods of analysis
c) Purity criteria
d) All of the above

6. The term "official" in relation to a drug in a pharmacopoeia means:
a) It is the most commonly used drug
b) It meets the standards set by the pharmacopoeia
c) It is approved by the FDA
d) It is available over-the-counter

7. Which of the following is NOT typically found in a pharmacopoeia?
a) Drug interactions
b) Analytical methods
c) Storage conditions
d) Impurity limits

8. The harmonization of pharmacopoeial standards globally is primarily coordinated by:
a) The International Conference on Harmonisation (ICH)
b) The World Health Organization (WHO)
c) The Pharmacopoeial Discussion Group (PDG)
d) The International Pharmaceutical Federation (FIP)

9. Which of the following is a key difference between a pharmacopoeia and a formulary?
a) A pharmacopoeia focuses on drug standards, while a formulary lists approved drugs for use
b) A pharmacopoeia is used internationally, while a formulary is only used nationally
c) A pharmacopoeia is updated annually, while a formulary is updated every decade
d) A pharmacopoeia is used by pharmacists, while a formulary is used by physicians

10. The European Pharmacopoeia is published by:
    a) European Union
    b) European Medicines Agency
    c) Council of Europe
    d) World Health Organization
11. Which of the following is NOT a common section in a pharmacopoeial monograph?
    a) Definition
    b) Identification tests
    c) Clinical trials data
    d) Assay
12. The concept of "pharmacopoeial harmonization" aims to:
    a) Create a single global pharmacopoeia
    b) Eliminate differences between national pharmacopoeias
    c) Reduce duplication of work in setting standards
    d) Replace national pharmacopoeias with regional ones
13. Which of the following is a correct statement about pharmacopoeial standards?
    a) They are legally binding in most countries
    b) They are only recommendations
    c) They apply only to over-the-counter drugs
    d) They are set by pharmaceutical companies
14. The British Pharmacopoeia is published by:
    a) Royal Pharmaceutical Society
    b) Medicines and Healthcare products Regulatory Agency
    c) National Health Service
    d) British Medical Association
15. Which of the following is NOT a typical function of a pharmacopoeia?
    a) Setting standards for drug quality
    b) Providing analytical methods for drug testing

c) Approving new drugs for market
d) Specifying storage conditions for drugs

16. The United States Pharmacopeia is revised:
a) Annually
b) Every 5 years
c) Every 10 years
d) Continuously with periodic publications

17. Which of the following is an example of a regional pharmacopoeia?
a) British Pharmacopoeia
b) European Pharmacopoeia
c) United States Pharmacopeia
d) Japanese Pharmacopoeia

18. The term "compendial" refers to:
a) Drugs listed in a pharmacopoeia
b) Drugs approved by regulatory agencies
c) Drugs manufactured by specific companies
d) Drugs used in compounding

19. Which of the following is NOT typically included in pharmacopoeial standards for a drug substance?
a) Description
b) Solubility
c) Marketing strategy
d) Related substances

20. The primary goal of pharmacopoeial harmonization is to:
a) Create uniform drug pricing globally
b) Establish consistent quality standards across different regions
c) Promote the use of generic drugs
d) Increase competition among drug manufacturers.

List of Important Questions

1. What is a pharmacopoeia, and what is its primary purpose?
2. How do pharmacopoeias contribute to ensuring drug quality and safety?
3. Describe the historical development of pharmacopoeias.
4. What are the main differences between national and international pharmacopoeias?
5. How often are pharmacopoeias typically updated, and why is this important?
6. What is the significance of the United States Pharmacopeia (USP) in global pharmaceutical standards?
7. Describe the structure and organization of a typical pharmacopoeia monograph.
8. How do pharmacopoeias address the issue of herbal medicines and traditional remedies?
9. What is the role of pharmacopoeias in setting standards for pharmaceutical excipients?
10. How do pharmacopoeias contribute to the harmonization of global pharmaceutical standards?
11. What are the key differences between a pharmacopoeia and a formulary?
12. How do pharmacopoeias address the quality control of biologics and biotechnology products?
13. What is the significance of reference standards provided by pharmacopoeias?
14. How do pharmacopoeias contribute to the fight against counterfeit medicines?
15. What are the challenges in maintaining and updating pharmacopoeias in the modern pharmaceutical landscape?

Bibliography

1. Wills S. Drugs of abuse. 2nd ed. London: Pharmaceutical Press; 2005.
2. Gaedcke F, Steinhoff B. Herbal medicinal products. Stuttgart: Medpharm Scientific Publishers; 2003.
3. Srivastava S, Mishra N. Genetic markers – a cutting-edge technology in herbal drug research. J Chem Pharm Res. 2009;1(1):1-18.
4. British Pharmacopoeia Commission. British pharmacopoeia 2019. London: TSO; 2018.
5. United States Pharmacopeial Convention. United States pharmacopeia and national formulary (USP 42-NF 37). Rockville, MD: United States Pharmacopeial Convention; 2019.
6. European Directorate for the Quality of Medicines & HealthCare. European pharmacopoeia. 10th ed. Strasbourg: Council of Europe; 2019.
7. World Health Organization. The international pharmacopoeia. 9th ed. Geneva: World Health Organization; 2019.
8. Japanese Pharmacopoeia Editorial Committee. The Japanese pharmacopoeia. 17th ed. Tokyo: Society of Japanese Pharmacopoeia; 2016.
9. Pharmacopoeia of the People's Republic of China. 2015 ed. Beijing: China Medical Science Press; 2015.
10. Singh H. Pharmacopoeias and formularies. In: A history of pharmacy in India and related aspects. Delhi: Vallabh Prakashan; 2002. p. 177-218.

CHAPTER 3

PACKAGING MATERIALS

Author

Dr. Pavan Kumar Yanamadala
Associate Professor, Department of Pharmacy Practice, Aditya Pharmacy College (A), Surampalem, Andhra Pradesh, India

Abstract

Packaging materials are crucial components in pharmaceutical products, serving multiple functions beyond mere containment. They protect drugs from environmental factors such as light, moisture, and oxygen, thereby preserving their stability and efficacy. Various materials are employed in pharmaceutical packaging, including glass, plastics, metals, and flexible laminates, each with specific properties suited to different drug formulations and dosage forms. Primary packaging, which comes into direct contact with the drug, requires careful selection to ensure compatibility and stability. Secondary and tertiary packaging provide additional protection and facilitate handling and distribution. The choice of packaging material considers factors such as moisture permeability, light transmission, gas barrier properties, and chemical inertness. Child-resistant and tamper-evident features are incorporated to enhance safety and prevent misuse. Environmental concerns have led to increased focus on sustainable packaging solutions, including recyclable and biodegradable materials. Innovative packaging technologies, such as active packaging and smart packaging, are emerging to improve drug stability and patient compliance. Regulatory requirements govern aspects of pharmaceutical packaging, including material selection, labeling, and testing standards, ensuring the safety and quality of packaged drug products throughout their shelf life.

Keywords: *Container closure system, Drug stability, Material compatibility, Barrier properties, Sustainability, Regulatory compliance*

Learning Objectives

After completion of the chapter, the student should be able to:

- Identify the various types of packaging materials used in pharmaceuticals.
- Explain the functions and requirements of pharmaceutical packaging.
- Describe the properties of different packaging materials (glass, plastic, metal, etc.).
- Evaluate the compatibility of packaging materials with different pharmaceutical products.
- Discuss the importance of packaging in maintaining drug stability and shelf life.
- Analyze the environmental impact of pharmaceutical packaging materials.
- Explain the regulatory requirements for pharmaceutical packaging materials.

INTRODUCTION TO PHARMACEUTICAL PACKAGING

Pharmaceutical packaging is a critical component in the lifecycle of a drug product, playing a pivotal role in maintaining its safety, efficacy, and quality from the point of manufacture to the end-user. It is far more than a mere container for holding medicinal products; rather, it is an intricate system designed to protect, preserve, and in some cases, even enhance the therapeutic effectiveness of the drug it contains. The science and art of pharmaceutical packaging involve a deep understanding of material properties, drug stability, regulatory requirements, and patient needs.

The primary function of packaging is to shield the

pharmaceutical product from various environmental factors that could potentially degrade or contaminate it. These factors include light, temperature, moisture, atmospheric gases, particulate matter, and microorganisms. Additionally, packaging must protect the product from mechanical stresses encountered during transportation and handling, such as vibration, compression, shock, and abrasion.

Ideal Characteristics of Pharmaceutical Packaging

An ideal pharmaceutical package should possess a range of characteristics to fulfill its multifaceted role effectively. Firstly, it must provide a robust barrier against environmental hazards. This includes protection from light, which can cause photodegradation of sensitive compounds; temperature fluctuations, which can affect drug stability; moisture, which can lead to hydrolysis or microbial growth; and atmospheric gases, particularly oxygen, which can cause oxidation of susceptible drugs.

Secondly, the packaging must withstand various mechanical stresses. It should be resistant to vibration, which is particularly important for liquid formulations to prevent agitation and potential degradation. The package should also have sufficient compression strength to withstand stacking during storage and transportation. Shock resistance is crucial, especially for glass containers or fragile dosage forms, to prevent breakage. Resistance to puncture and abrasion ensures the integrity of the package is maintained throughout its lifecycle.

Thirdly, the ideal package must maintain the integrity of its contents. This means preventing both loss and gain of moisture, which is critical for maintaining the stability of hygroscopic drugs. It should also prevent the loss of volatile materials from the drug formulation. Importantly, the packaging material itself must not interact with the drug product – it should neither shed particles into the contents nor leach any substances that could contaminate or react with the drug.

The aesthetic aspect of packaging, while seemingly secondary, plays a significant role in the pharmaceutical market. An attractive and well-designed package can enhance patient compliance and brand recognition. However, this must be balanced with functionality – the package should be easy to label for clear identification and should facilitate ease of use for the patient.

From an economic and environmental perspective, the ideal pharmaceutical package should be cost-effective to produce while meeting all necessary quality standards. There is also an increasing emphasis on the use of biodegradable or recyclable materials to minimize environmental impact.

Levels of Packaging

Pharmaceutical packaging is typically divided into three levels:

1. Primary Packaging: This is the packaging in direct contact with the drug product. Examples include blister packs, vials, ampoules, and bottles. Primary packaging must be compatible with the drug and provide the first line of defense against environmental factors.
2. Secondary Packaging: This contains the primary packaged product. It typically includes cartons or boxes that hold one or more units of the primary package. Secondary packaging provides additional protection and is where most of the product information and branding are displayed.
3. Tertiary Packaging: This is used for bulk handling, warehouse storage, and shipping. It includes larger containers like corrugated boxes

or barrels that contain multiple units of secondary packaging.

Pharmaceutical packaging must comply with various regulatory guidelines to ensure product safety and quality. These include:

1. Good Manufacturing Practices (GMP): Packaging operations must adhere to GMP guidelines to ensure consistent quality and safety.
2. Pharmacopoeial Standards: Many pharmacopoeias, such as the United States Pharmacopeia (USP) and European Pharmacopoeia (Ph. Eur.), provide standards for packaging materials and container closure systems.
3. Environmental Regulations: There is increasing pressure to use environmentally friendly packaging materials and designs.
4. Child-Resistant and Senior-Friendly Packaging: Many jurisdictions require certain medications to be packaged in containers that are difficult for children to open but still accessible for elderly patients.

Current Trends in Pharmaceutical Packaging

The field of pharmaceutical packaging continues to evolve, driven by technological advancements and changing market demands. Some emerging trends include:

1. Smart Packaging: This involves the integration of technologies like RFID (Radio-Frequency Identification) tags for tracking and anti-counterfeiting measures. Some smart packaging can even monitor environmental conditions or patient adherence.
2. Sustainable Packaging: There is a growing focus

on developing eco-friendly materials and designs to reduce the environmental impact of pharmaceutical packaging.

3. Patient-Centric Packaging: Designs that improve adherence and ease of use, particularly for patients with physical limitations or complex medication regimens.
4. Personalized Packaging: As personalized medicine advances, there may be a need for more flexible, small-batch packaging solutions.

Types of Packaging Materials

Packaging materials play a crucial role in protecting and preserving pharmaceutical products. The main types of materials used for containers and closures include glass, metals, plastics, and rubber. Glass is categorized into various types, such as borosilicate, treated soda-lime, regular soda-lime, general-purpose soda-lime, and colored glass. Metals like tin, iron, aluminum, and lead are also used in packaging. Plastics are divided into thermosetting resins (phenolics and urea) and thermoplastic resins (including polyethylene, polypropylene, PVC, polystyrene, polycarbonate, polyamide, acrylic multipolymers, and PET). Rubber, both natural and synthetic varieties like neoprene and butyl rubber, is another important packaging material.

Selection Criteria of Packaging Material

When selecting packaging materials for pharmaceutical products, several crucial factors must be considered. The chosen materials should effectively protect the preparation from environmental conditions while remaining non-reactive with the product. It's essential that the packaging does not impart any tastes or odors to the contents and is non-toxic. Additionally, the materials must be FDA-approved and meet applicable tamper-resistance requirements. Practical considerations include adaptability to high-speed packaging equipment and reasonable cost relative to the product value. These criteria ensure that the packaging not only preserves the product's integrity but also meets regulatory standards and practical manufacturing needs.

Glass

Glass is a versatile and widely used packaging material in the pharmaceutical industry. It is primarily composed of sand (silica), soda-ash (sodium carbonate), and limestone (calcium carbonate). The properties of glass can be modified by adding various oxides, such as sodium oxide, calcium oxide, or boron oxide. Pure silica glass has a rigid network structure, making it hard and chemically resistant but difficult to mold due to its high melting point. The addition of sodium oxide reduces the melting point but increases water reactivity. Calcium oxide and similar divalent oxides increase rigidity and chemical resistance. Boron or aluminum oxides create a flexible yet chemically resistant structure. These variations in composition result in different types of glass suitable for various pharmaceutical applications..

Table: Types of glass

The pharmaceutical industry utilizes several types of glass, each with specific properties and applications. Type I Borosilicate glass, known for its high chemical resistance and low leaching, is ideal for laboratory apparatus and injections. Type II Treated soda-lime glass, with its water-resistant surface, is suitable for alkali-sensitive products and large volume containers. Type III Regular soda-lime glass is used for solid dosage forms and oily injections but not for aqueous or alkali-sensitive drugs. Type NP glass is designated for non-parenteral use in oral and topical preparations. Neutral glass, with its softness and autoclave resistance, is used for small vials and large transfusion bottles. Neutral tubing for ampoules has a lower melting point, making it easy to seal. Colored glass, particularly amber, is used for photosensitive products as it resists UV and visible radiation

Advantages and Disadvantages of glass containers

Glass containers offer numerous advantages in pharmaceutical packaging. They are strong, rigid, and transparent, allowing for visual inspection of contents. Their availability in various shapes and sizes adds to their versatility. Borosilicate and neutral glasses are heat-resistant, facilitating sterilization. Glass is chemically inert, especially in borosilicate and treated soda-lime varieties, and can be customized by altering its composition. It's also cost-effective and doesn't deteriorate with age when properly sealed. However, glass containers do have some drawbacks. They are brittle and susceptible to breakage, especially with sudden temperature changes. They're heavier than plastic alternatives and, unless colored, allow UV light passage, which can be detrimental to photosensitive drugs. Some types of glass may experience flaking or weathering, which can compromise the integrity of the contents

PLASTICS

Plastics are synthetic polymers widely used in pharmaceutical packaging due to their versatile properties. They are generally heat-sensitive, with many types melting or softening at relatively low temperatures. However, some plastics like nylon, polycarbonate, polypropylene, and high-density polyethylene can withstand autoclaving. Plastic containers are lightweight, mechanically strong, and resistant to inorganic chemicals, though they may be vulnerable to organic solvents and oils. One concern with plastics is the potential for additives to contaminate the contents. Additionally, most plastics are not completely impermeable to water vapor and gases. Plastics are classified into thermoplastic types, which soften when heated and harden upon cooling, and thermosetting types, which maintain their shape until decomposition due to high cross-linking

GLASS TRANSITION TEMPERATURE (T_g)

The glass transition temperature (Tg) is a critical property of plastics, defining the point below which they become rigid and brittle. Above Tg, thermoplastics soften and eventually melt, while thermosetting plastics may decompose before softening due to their high degree of cross-linking. To enhance stability and performance, various additives are incorporated into plastics. These include stabilizers to prevent side reactions, antioxidants to combat oxidation, pigments for decoration and UV protection, fillers for cost reduction and performance enhancement, and plasticizers to reduce Tg. Other additives such as cross-linking agents, curing agents, activators, and accelerators may also be used to achieve specific properties in the final plastic product.

PLASTIC MATERIALS

Table 3.2: Types of plastics

Material and uses	**Pros**	**Cons**
HDPE (ϱ=0.955) Uses: Detergents, bleaches, milk, foods, drugs, cosmetics	Inert, cheap, low water vapor transmission, tough	Semi-opaque, taste transfer, absorbs solutions
LDPE (ϱ=0.920) Uses: Cosmetics, personal products, foods	Squeezable, inert, cheap	Poor barrier for non-polar molecules, high water vapor transmission
Polystyrene (ϱ=1.05) Uses: Dry drugs, petroleum jelly	Clear, stiff, cheap	High water vapor transmission, crack-prone, poor impact
Rigid PVC (ϱ=1.35) Uses: Shampoo, bath oil, detergent	Clear, stiff, O2-barrier, retains non-polar molecules	Many additives, hard to process, solvent-sensitive
Polypropylene (ϱ=0.90)	Inert, cheap	Brittle at low temps, high stabilizer content
Polyamide (ϱ=1.10) Uses: Foods, drugs, cosmetics, aerosols	Good barrier, tough, O2-barrier, sterilizable	Expensive, absorbs water

Material and uses	**Pros**	**Cons**
Polycarbonate (ϱ=1.20) Uses: Drugs, cosmetics	Very tough, clear, sterilizable	Expensive, solvent-sensitive, poor water/O2 barrier
PMMA (ϱ=1.10) Uses: Drugs, cosmetics	Clear, good for oils	Poor water vapor and O2 barrier
PET Uses: Carbonated/mineral waters, mouthwashes, cosmetics	Strong, good gas and aroma barrier	-

Structures of some common plastics

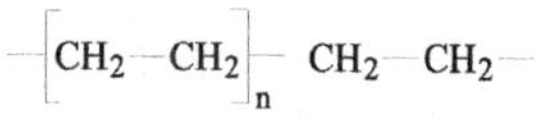

Polyethylene (T_g = – 120°C)

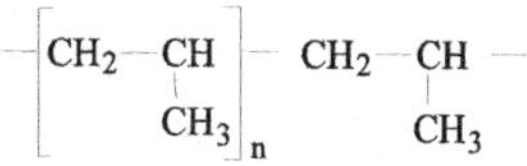

Polypropylene (T_g = – 27°C)

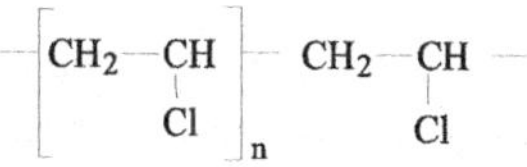

Polyvinylchloride ,PVC (T_g = 80°C)

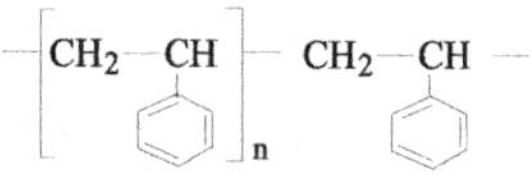

Polystyrene (T_g = 100°C)

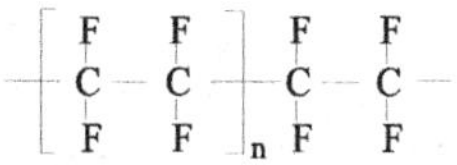

Polytetrafluroethylene (T_g = 126°C)

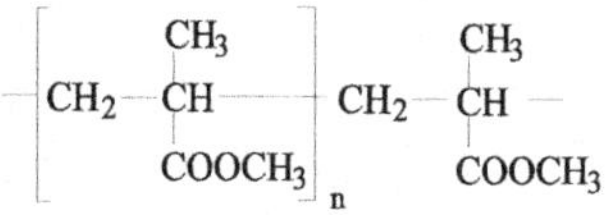

Polymethylmethacrylate, PMMA (T_g = 110°C)

Thermosetting plastics

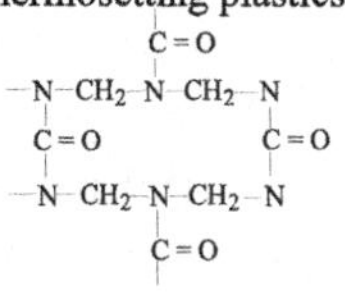

Urea formaldehyde

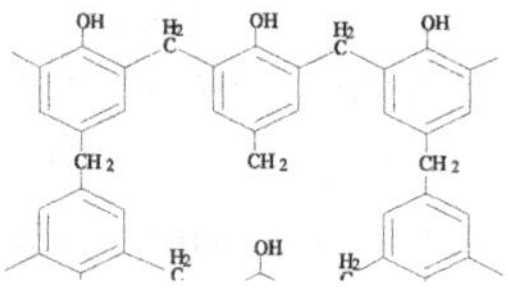

Phenol formaldehyde

DRUG-PLASTIC CONSIDERATION

The interaction between drugs and plastic packaging is a critical aspect of pharmaceutical product design. These interactions are categorized into five main areas: permeation, leaching, sorption, chemical reaction, and alteration in the physical properties of plastics or products. Each of these categories presents unique challenges that can affect the stability, efficacy, and safety of drug products.

Permeation

Permeation involves the transmission of gases, vapors, or liquids through plastic packaging materials. This process can significantly impact a drug's shelf life. For instance, the permeation of water vapor and oxygen through plastic walls can be problematic for drugs sensitive to hydrolysis and oxidation. The extent of permeation is influenced by factors such as temperature and humidity. Different plastics have varying permeability properties; for example, nylons are poor barriers for water due to their hydrophilic nature, while hydrophobic materials like polyethylene provide better protection. Volatile ingredients in formulations may permeate through container walls, potentially altering the aroma of cosmetics or the taste of medicinal products. In some cases, specific components of formulations, such as the oil phase in water-in-oil emulsions, may migrate into hydrophobic plastic containers.

Leaching

Leaching refers to the migration of additives from plastic packaging into the drug product. This can lead to contamination of the drug and potentially toxic effects, especially if dyes or other harmful substances leach into parenteral solutions. In some cases, leached components may catalyze reactions in the solution, leading to drug decomposition. The risk of leaching necessitates careful selection of plastic materials and additives for pharmaceutical packaging.

Sorption

Sorption involves the removal of constituents from the drug product by the packaging material. This process can be particularly problematic for high-potency drugs administered in small doses, where even minor losses can significantly affect therapeutic efficacy. A common issue is the loss of preservatives, which can leave products vulnerable to microbial growth. Factors influencing sorption include the chemical structure of the solute, pH, solvent system, concentration of solute, temperature, contact time, and contact area. Understanding these factors is crucial for minimizing sorption-related issues in drug packaging.

Chemical Reactivity

Chemical reactions can occur between components of the plastic packaging and ingredients in the drug formulation. Even trace amounts of chemically incompatible substances can alter the appearance or properties of the plastic or the drug product. This reactivity underscores the importance of thorough compatibility testing between packaging materials and drug formulations.

Modification

Modification refers to physical and chemical alterations of the packaging material caused by the drug product. For example, polyethylene containers may deform due to gas permeation or content loss through container walls. Certain substances can have specific effects on plastics: oils can soften polyethylene and PVC, while fluorinated hydrocarbons may attack these materials. In some cases, the drug product might extract plasticizers, antioxidants, or stabilizers from the plastic, altering its flexibility. Conversely, the extraction of plasticizers by solvents can make container walls stiffer.

These drug-plastic considerations highlight the complexity of selecting appropriate packaging materials for pharmaceutical products. Manufacturers must carefully evaluate these potential interactions to ensure the stability, safety, and efficacy of their products throughout their intended shelf life. This often involves extensive compatibility testing and may require the use of specialized packaging materials or protective measures to mitigate these issues

METALS

Tin

Tin stands out for its exceptional resistance to chemical attack, making it an ideal choice for pharmaceutical packaging. Its ability to coat other metals enhances their properties, as seen in tin-coated lead tubes that combine lead's malleability with tin's chemical inertness. This combination was particularly useful in packaging fluoride toothpaste in the past.

Despite its advantages, tin's higher cost compared to other metals like lead, aluminium, and iron is a significant drawback. Nevertheless, its benefits often outweigh this limitation in specific applications. Tin containers are favored for food packaging, particularly for products like milk powder. In the pharmaceutical industry, some eye ointments continue to be packaged in pure tin tubes, showcasing the metal's ongoing relevance in certain niche applications.

Aluminium

Aluminium offers a compelling set of advantages for pharmaceutical packaging. Its light weight significantly reduces shipping costs, making it an economical choice for large-scale distribution. Aluminium packaging provides an appealing aesthetic similar to tin but at a lower cost, making it an attractive option for manufacturers.

One of aluminium's most notable features is its ability to form a thin, transparent oxide coating upon exposure to atmospheric oxygen. This natural barrier protects the metal from further oxidation, enhancing its durability. However, this protective layer is susceptible to substances with high or low pH levels and certain complexing agents, which can lead to corrosion. In some cases, this corrosion process may result in hydrogen gas evolution, which can be problematic for certain pharmaceutical products.

Aluminium finds widespread use in the pharmaceutical industry, including ointment tubes, screw caps, and strip packaging for tablets and capsules. To mitigate potential reactions with package contents, internally lacquered aluminium containers are sometimes employed.

Iron

While pure iron is rarely used in pharmaceutical packaging, tin-coated steel (commonly referred to as 'tin') is prevalent. This material combines the strength of steel with tin's corrosion resistance, offering a robust packaging solution. However, it's important to note that if an aqueous liquid penetrates a fault in the tin layer, it can create a galvanic cell, leading to rapid corrosion of the underlying steel. To combat this issue, the tin surface is often lacquered for additional protection.

Tin-coated steel is widely used in the fabrication of

milk containers, screw caps, and aerosol cans, demonstrating its versatility in both food and pharmaceutical packaging.

Lead

Lead offers the advantage of being the least expensive metal used in pharmaceutical containers. Its malleability makes it easy to work with and shape into various forms. However, the risk of lead poisoning when ingested poses a significant health hazard, severely limiting its use in pharmaceutical packaging.

To mitigate this risk, lead containers and tubes must always have an internal lining of an inert metal or polymer. With proper lining, lead tubes can be safely used for products such as fluoride toothpaste. However, due to increasing awareness of lead's toxicity, its use in pharmaceutical packaging has significantly decreased over time, with safer alternatives being preferred in most applications.

RUBBER

Natural rubber is a remarkable material composed of long-chain polymers of isoprene units linked in the cis-position. The primary source of this versatile substance is the *Hevea braziliensis* tree, which produces a latex containing 30-40% rubber in colloidal suspension when its bark is carefully incised.

Two main methods are employed to prepare solid rubbers from this latex:

Smoked Sheet

This process involves coagulating the negatively charged rubber particles by adding small amounts of acetic or formic acid. The resulting spongy mass is rolled into sheets, washed, and then smoked over a wood fire. The phenolic compounds from the smoke not only impart a brown color but also act as preservatives, protecting the rubber from mold growth. However, due to the presence of non-rubber materials, smoked sheet rubber is generally not used for pharmaceutical purposes.

Pale Crepe

This method produces a purer form of rubber suitable for pharmaceutical applications. The coagulated rubber is thoroughly washed and then repeatedly squeezed between rollers while being sprayed with water. This process removes most non-rubber constituents, resulting in a cleaner, pale-colored product.

Compounding Rubbers

Raw rubber, while useful, has limitations such as poor elasticity and sensitivity to temperature changes. To enhance its properties and make it suitable for a wide range of applications, various additives are incorporated:

Vulcanizing Agents

Sulfur is commonly used to create cross-links between rubber molecules, dramatically improving elasticity, strength, and temperature resistance. Vulcanization can be achieved through heat treatment or cold curing with sulfur monochloride.

Accelerators

These compounds, such as 2-mercapto benzthiazol (MBT) and tetramethyl thiuram disulfide (TMT), reduce vulcanization time and sulfur requirements.

Activators: Substances like stearic acid or zinc oxide enhance the effectiveness of accelerators.

Fillers: Both reinforcing fillers (e.g., carbon black, zinc oxide) and extending fillers (e.g., talc) are used to improve physical properties and reduce costs.

Softeners

Additives like pine oil or mineral oil facilitate the incorporation of fillers and ease manufacturing.

Antioxidants

Compounds such as phenyl betanaphthyl amine protect against oxidative degradation.

Pigments and Lubricants: These are added for coloration and to assist in molding processes, respectively.

Synthetic Rubbers

Several synthetic rubbers have been developed to address specific needs in pharmaceutical packaging:

Butyl Rubber

This copolymer of isobutylene and isoprene offers excellent resistance to aging and chemical attack, low permeability to water vapor and air, and low water absorption. However, it has limited oil and solvent resistance and begins to decompose at high temperatures.

Nitrile Rubber

Known for its oil and heat resistance, nitrile rubber does have the drawback of potentially absorbing bactericides and leaching extractives.

Chloroprene Rubber (Neoprene)

This polymer offers good aging properties, oil resistance, and heat stability. It also has lower water absorption and permeability compared to natural rubber.

Silicone Rubber

While expensive, silicone rubber boasts excellent heat

resistance, extremely low water absorption and permeability, and outstanding aging characteristics. However, it has poor tensile strength

PHARMACEUTICAL PACKAGES

1. CONTAINERS

In the pharmaceutical industry, containers play a crucial role in preserving the integrity, safety, and efficacy of drug products. The choice of container is based on the specific requirements of the drug, its form, and intended use. Here's an overview of various types of pharmaceutical containers and their applications:

Types of Containers Based on Closure and Use

1. Well-closed Containers:
   These containers protect the preparation from external solid contaminants and prevent content loss during handling, storage, and transport. They are suitable for products that don't require stringent protection from atmospheric conditions.
2. Airtight Containers:
   Designed to shield the contents from atmospheric contamination by liquids, solids, or vapors, these containers are crucial for drugs susceptible to efflorescence, deliquescence, evaporation, or oxidation.
3. Hermetically Sealed Containers: These containers, such as glass ampoules sealed by fusion, provide an impermeable barrier to air and other gases, offering the highest level of protection.
4. Light-resistant Containers: Used for photosensitive drugs, these containers are

typically made of amber-colored glass or opaque materials to prevent light-induced decomposition.

5. Single-dose Containers: These containers, like ampoules, are designed to deliver a single dose of medication, ensuring precise dosage and minimizing contamination risks.
6. Multi-dose Containers: These containers, such as vials, hold multiple doses of a drug and are designed for repeated use while maintaining the product's integrity.
7. Aerosol Containers: Specially designed to withstand internal pressure, these containers are used for products delivered as fine mists or sprays.

Container Types Based on Shape and Material

Glass/Polyethylene Bottles:

- Narrow-mouth bottles are used for low-viscosity liquids like gargles and elixirs.
- Wide-mouth bottles are preferred for solids (powders, tablets) and high-viscosity liquids or suspensions.
- Colored, fluted bottles are used for external-use preparations to distinguish them from internal-use products.

Dropper Bottles/Droptainers:

These are used for dispensing eye drops, ear drops, and nasal drops. Modern plastic droptainers combine the bottle and dropper in a single, squeezable unit.

Collapsible Tubes

Made of plastic or metal, these are used for semi-solid preparations like ointments, pastes, and gels.

Ampoules:

Made from low-melting-point neutral glass, these single-dose containers are heat-sealed to ensure sterility.

Vials: Used for multi-dose injectable preparations, these containers feature a rubber closure that can be pierced by a needle while maintaining the sterility of the contents.

Polyethylene Packets for Infusion Fluids: Flexible bags made of PVC, polyethylene, or polypropylene are increasingly used for intravenous fluids, offering advantages in storage and administration.

Glass Bottles for IV Fluids: Traditionally used for intravenous solutions, these are being gradually replaced by flexible plastic bags.

Aerosol Containers: Designed to withstand high pressure, these containers are used for products delivered as sprays or foams

CLOSURE AND CLOSURE LINERS

Closures are integral components of pharmaceutical packaging, serving as barriers between the product and the external environment. They play a crucial role in maintaining product integrity, preventing contamination, and ensuring safety. The pharmaceutical industry utilizes various closure designs, each tailored to specific product requirements and user needs.

1. Screw-On Closures: Screw-on closures, including threaded caps and lug caps, are widely used in the pharmaceutical industry. Threaded caps engage with corresponding threads on the

container neck, while lug caps use interrupted threads for quicker opening. These closures are typically made from metals like aluminum or tinplate, or plastics such as polypropylene or high-density polyethylene. Metal caps often feature an internal enamel or lacquer coating to prevent corrosion and product interaction.

2. Crimp-On Closures: Crown caps, a common type of crimp-on closure, are primarily used for glass bottles. These metal caps are crimped onto the bottle's lip, creating a tight seal. While less common in pharmaceuticals, they may be used for certain liquid formulations.
3. Press-On Closures: Also known as snap caps, these closures rely on friction and a slight interference fit to stay in place. They're often used for over-the-counter products where ease of opening is desirable.
4. Roll-On Closures: These closures start as smooth metal shells that are placed on threaded bottle necks. The threading is then formed by rolling or pressing the shell onto the bottle. This method accommodates slight variations in glass bottle dimensions, making it particularly suitable for large-scale production.
5. Pilfer-Proof Closures: A variation of roll-on closures, these feature an extended skirt that breaks away from the main cap upon first opening, providing evidence of tampering. They're commonly used in pharmaceutical and nutraceutical products to enhance safety and consumer confidence.

Closure Liners

Closure liners are essential for creating an effective

seal between the closure and the container. They prevent leakage, protect against contamination, and can provide additional barrier properties.

Types of Liners:

1. Homogeneous Liners: Single-material liners, often in disk or ring form. They provide uniform properties and can withstand high-temperature sterilization, making them suitable for many pharmaceutical applications.
2. Heterogeneous or Composite Liners: Multi-layered liners combining different materials to meet specific requirements. Typically, they consist of a facing (in contact with the product) and a backing (providing cushioning and sealing properties).

Key Considerations for Liner Selection:

- Chemical compatibility with the product
- Barrier properties against moisture and gases
- Heat resistance for sterilization processes
- Torque requirements for opening and resealing
- Shelf-life stability
- Cost-effectiveness

Tamper-Resistant Packaging

Tamper-resistant packaging has become increasingly important in the pharmaceutical industry, especially for over-the-counter products. These systems provide visible evidence of any attempt to access the product before purchase.

FDA-Approved Tamper-Resistant Packaging Systems:

1. Film Wrappers:

   a) End-folded wrapper: Utilizes heat-sealed, gift-wrap style folding.

   b) Fin seal wrapper: Creates a crimped seal

between two film surfaces.
c) Shrink wrapper: Uses heat-shrinkable films to tightly encase the product.

2. Blister Packages:
   Formed by vacuum-drawing thermoplastic sheets into molds, then sealing with a backing material. Common materials include PVC, PVC/PE combinations, and high-barrier laminates for moisture-sensitive products.
3. Strip Packages:
   Created by sealing products between two layers of flexible film. Ideal for unit-dose packaging of tablets and capsules.
4. Aerosol Containers:
   Typically made of drawn aluminum with specialized coatings for product compatibility. These containers use a combination of product and propellant, sealed with a crimped spray nozzle and valve assembly.
5. Other Systems:
   - Bubble packs
   - Shrink seals and bands
   - Foil, paper, or plastic pouches
   - Bottle seals and tape seals
   - Breakable caps
   - Sealed tubes and cartons

The choice of tamper-resistant packaging depends on the product characteristics, regulatory requirements, and consumer usability considerations. Many of these systems not only provide tamper evidence but also offer additional benefits such as moisture protection, light resistance, and enhanced product stability.

EVALUATION OF PACKAGING MATERIALS

The evaluation of packaging materials is a critical process in the pharmaceutical industry, ensuring that the chosen materials maintain the safety, stability, and efficacy of drug products throughout their shelf life. Different types of packaging materials undergo specific tests to assess their suitability for pharmaceutical use. This comprehensive overview delves into the evaluation methods for various packaging materials, highlighting their importance in maintaining product integrity.

A. Glass Containers

Glass containers are widely used in the pharmaceutical industry due to their inert nature and excellent barrier properties. However, even the highest quality pharmaceutical glass is not entirely free from extractable alkali, necessitating specific tests to ensure their suitability.

Test for Hydrolytic Resistance (Limit of Alkalinity)

This test is fundamental in assessing the quality of glass containers. It is performed using two main methods: the crushed glass test and the whole container test.

The crushed glass test is applicable to all types of glass containers except surface-treated glass (Type II). In this test, the container is crushed and sieved to produce a uniform particle size. A specific weight of this glass powder is then autoclaved with a measured amount of distilled water. After cooling and filtration, the extract is titrated with standard sulfuric acid. This method ensures that a constant surface area of glass is exposed to the solution, providing consistent results.

For surface-treated glass containers (Type II), the whole container test is employed. In this method, intact containers are filled with distilled water and subjected to autoclaving conditions. The extracts from several containers are pooled and titrated with standard hydrochloric acid, as per Indian Pharmacopoeia guidelines.

The limits for alkalinity vary depending on the type of glass. Type I glass, which is highly resistant borosilicate glass, has the strictest limit of 1.0 ml of 0.05 N sulfuric acid per 10g of glass. Type II glass, treated soda-lime glass, has limits of 0.7 ml for containers up to 100 ml and 0.2 ml for larger containers. Type III soda-lime glass has a higher limit of 8.5 ml, while general-purpose soda-lime glass (N.P.) has the highest limit of 15.0 ml.

B. Metal Containers for Eye Ointments

Metal collapsible tubes, commonly used for eye ointments, undergo rigorous testing for metal particles. This test is crucial to ensure that no metal particles contaminate the ointment, which could cause serious eye irritation or damage.

The test procedure involves filling empty tubes with an ointment base and sealing them overnight. The ointment is then squeezed through a heated metal bacteriological filter assembly fitted with a suitable filter paper. After washing the filter paper with chloroform and drying it, it is examined under a magnifying glass with oblique light.

The observed metal particles are categorized based on their size, and a scoring system is applied. Particles 1 mm and above receive 50 points, those between 0.5 mm and 1 mm receive 10 points, particles between 0.2 mm and 0.5 mm receive 2 points, and those less than 0.2 mm receive no points. The lot of tubes passes the test if the total score is less than 100 points for 50 tubes. If the score is between 100 and 150, the test is repeated with 50 more tubes, and the lot passes if the total for 100 tubes is less than 150 points.

C. Plastic Containers

Plastic containers have gained popularity in pharmaceutical packaging due to their versatility and cost-effectiveness. However, they must undergo a series of tests to ensure their suitability for pharmaceutical use.

The leakage test is performed by filling ten containers with water, fitting them with closures, and keeping them inverted at room temperature for 24 hours. This test ensures the integrity of the container and closure system, as any signs of leakage would render the containers unsuitable for use.

For containers designed to be squeezed, such as those for creams or ointments, a collapsibility test is conducted. This test ensures that the container, when collapsed inwards during use, yields at least 90% of its nominal contents at the required rate of flow at ambient temperature.

The transparency test is crucial for containers where visual inspection of the contents is necessary. A diluted standard suspension is prepared, and containers are filled with this suspension. The contents should be detectable when viewed through the containers, compared to containers filled with water.

Water vapor permeability is assessed by filling containers with water, sealing them, and monitoring weight loss over 14 days under controlled temperature and humidity conditions. The loss in weight should not exceed 0.2%, ensuring that the containers provide adequate protection against moisture loss or gain.

Additional tests for plastic containers include analysis for heavy metals such as barium, tin, and zinc. Extraction tests are also performed, where a specified surface area of the plastic is extracted with a suitable medium. The extract is then subjected to various tests including appearance assessment, light absorption measurement, determination of non-volatile matter and residue on ignition, heavy metal analysis, buffering capacity evaluation, and testing for oxidizable substances.

Bacteriological tests are equally important, involving the injection or instillation of specific extracts from the material into animals to determine their biological response. This helps ensure that the plastic material does not elicit any adverse biological reactions when in contact with pharmaceutical products or body tissues

Summary

Packaging materials form the crucial interface between pharmaceutical products and the external environment, playing a multifaceted role in preserving drug integrity, ensuring safety, and facilitating proper use. Primary packaging materials, in direct contact with the drug, include glass, plastics, metals, and rubber, each selected based on their unique properties and compatibility with specific dosage forms. Glass, with its excellent chemical resistance and impermeability, remains a preferred choice for many liquid formulations and some solid dosage forms. Various types of glass, from Type I borosilicate to Type III soda-lime glass, are employed based on the drug's sensitivity and intended use. Plastics offer versatility and have gained prominence due to their light weight and shatter resistance. Polymers like polyethylene, polypropylene, and polyvinyl chloride find extensive use in bottles, blister packs, and flexible containers, with their selection guided by factors such as moisture barrier properties and drug compatibility. Metals, particularly aluminum, are utilized in blister packaging and tubes, prized for their excellent barrier properties against light, moisture, and gases. Rubber closures, critical for injectable products, undergo rigorous testing to ensure they don't leach substances or adsorb drug components. The selection of packaging materials involves careful consideration of drug-package interactions, environmental protection needs, and stability requirements throughout the product's shelf life. Advanced packaging technologies, including active packaging with oxygen scavengers or desiccants, and intelligent packaging incorporating time-temperature indicators, represent cutting-edge solutions for enhancing product stability and monitoring. Secondary packaging elements like cartons and labels play vital roles in product identification, tamper-evidence, and conveying crucial information to users. The regulatory landscape surrounding pharmaceutical packaging is complex, encompassing good manufacturing practices, stability testing protocols, and labeling requirements. Environmental considerations have gained prominence, driving trends towards sustainable and eco-friendly packaging solutions. Quality control of packaging materials involves a battery of tests, from physical and chemical analyses to performance evaluations, ensuring consistent quality and safeguarding the drug product throughout its lifecycle.

Multiple Choice Questions

1. Which of the following is NOT a primary function of pharmaceutical packaging?
   a) Protection
   b) Containment
   c) Drug synthesis
   d) Information
2. Which packaging material is most commonly used for tablets and capsules?
   a) Glass
   b) Plastic
   c) Metal
   d) Paper
3. The term "barrier properties" in packaging refers to:
   a) Physical strength of the package
   b) Resistance to moisture and gas permeation
   c) Ability to withstand high temperatures
   d) Resistance to light penetration
4. Which type of glass is preferred for packaging parenteral preparations?
   a) Soda-lime glass
   b) Borosilicate glass
   c) Lead glass
   d) Fused silica glass
5. Which plastic is commonly used for making squeeze bottles for liquid medications?
   a) Polyethylene
   b) Polystyrene
   c) Polyvinyl chloride
   d) Polypropylene
6. The process of coating the inner surface of a glass container with silicon dioxide is known as:
   a) Siliconization
   b) Lamination

c) Annealing
d) Tempering

7. Which of the following is an advantage of plastic packaging over glass?
a) Better barrier properties
b) Higher transparency
c) Lighter weight
d) Better chemical inertness

8. Blister packs are typically made of:
a) Aluminum foil and plastic film
b) Paper and wax
c) Glass and metal
d) Rubber and plastic

9. Which of the following is NOT a common type of closure for pharmaceutical containers?
a) Screw cap
b) Flip-top cap
c) Magnetic cap
d) Child-resistant cap

10. The term "primary packaging" refers to:
a) The outermost layer of packaging
b) The packaging in direct contact with the product
c) The most expensive packaging component
d) The largest packaging component

11. Which of the following materials is commonly used for making collapsible tubes for ointments and creams?
a) Aluminum
b) Glass
c) Paper
d) Polyethylene

12. The process of treating glass containers to reduce surface alkalinity is called:
a) Annealing

b) Tempering
c) Sulfur treatment
d) Etching

13. Which type of plastic is known for its excellent barrier properties against moisture and gases?
a) Polyethylene
b) Polypropylene
c) Polyvinyl chloride
d) Polyvinylidene chloride

14. The term "unit dose packaging" refers to:
a) Packaging containing multiple doses of a drug
b) Packaging containing a single dose of a drug
c) Packaging used only in hospitals
d) Packaging for liquid medications

15. Which of the following is a advantage of aluminum foil in pharmaceutical packaging?
a) Transparency
b) Flexibility
c) Complete barrier to light and moisture
d) Low cost

16. The process of sealing a glass ampule is typically done by:
a) Heat sealing
b) Adhesive bonding
c) Mechanical crimping
d) Ultrasonic welding

17. Which type of packaging is commonly used for effervescent tablets?
a) Blister packs
b) Glass bottles
c) Aluminum tubes
d) Paper sachets

18. The term "secondary packaging" refers to:
a) Packaging that comes in direct contact with the drug

b) Packaging that contains the primary packaged product
c) Packaging used for transportation
d) Packaging used for display purposes

19. Which of the following is NOT a common test for evaluating the quality of pharmaceutical packaging materials?
a) Water vapor transmission rate
b) Light transmission
c) Tensile strength
d) Drug potency

20. The use of desiccants in pharmaceutical packaging is primarily to:
a) Enhance the flavor of the product
b) Absorb moisture
c) Prevent microbial growth
d) Improve the appearance of the package.

List of Important Questions

1. What are the primary functions of pharmaceutical packaging?
2. How does packaging contribute to the stability and shelf life of pharmaceutical products?
3. What are the main types of primary packaging materials used in pharmaceuticals?
4. Describe the advantages and disadvantages of glass as a packaging material for pharmaceuticals.
5. What are the key properties of plastic materials used in pharmaceutical packaging?
6. How do barrier properties of packaging materials affect drug stability?
7. What are the considerations for choosing packaging materials for liquid dosage forms?
8. Describe the types of closures used for pharmaceutical containers and their importance.
9. What are the unique packaging requirements for sterile pharmaceutical products?
10. How does packaging contribute to the prevention of counterfeiting in pharmaceuticals?
11. What are the environmental considerations in pharmaceutical packaging?
12. Describe the role of secondary and tertiary packaging in the pharmaceutical supply chain.
13. What are the regulatory requirements for pharmaceutical packaging materials?
14. How does packaging contribute to patient compliance and proper use of medications?
15. What are the latest innovations in smart packaging for pharmaceuticals?

Bibliography

1. Pilchik R. Pharmaceutical blister packaging, part I: Rationale and materials. Pharm Technol. 2000;24(11):68-78.
2. Lockhart H, Paine FA. Packaging of pharmaceuticals and healthcare products. London: Blackie Academic & Professional; 1996.
3. Dean DA, Evans ER, Hall IH. Pharmaceutical packaging technology. London: Taylor & Francis; 2000.
4. Bauer EJ. Pharmaceutical packaging handbook. New York: Informa Healthcare; 2009.
5. Pilchik R. Pharmaceutical blister packaging, part II: Machinery and assembly. Pharm Technol. 2000;24(12):56-60.
6. Forcinio H. Pharmaceutical packaging: Trends and innovations. Pharm Technol. 2019;43(4):20-7.
7. Yam KL, editor. The Wiley encyclopedia of packaging technology. 3rd ed. Hoboken: John Wiley & Sons; 2009.
8. Mehta RM. Pharmaceutics-I. 6th ed. Delhi: Vallabh Prakashan; 2016.
9. Coles R, McDowell D, Kirwan MJ, editors. Food packaging technology. Oxford: Blackwell Publishing; 2003.
10. Murthy PN, Sowjanya N. Pharmaceutical packaging: current trends and future. Int J Pharm Pharm Sci. 2014;6(6):480-5.

CHAPTER 4

PHARMACEUTICAL AIDS

Author

Mr. Anilkumar Vadaga

Associate Professor, GIET School of Pharmacy, Rajahmundry, Andhra Pradesh, India

Abstract

Pharmaceutical aids, also known as excipients, are essential components in drug formulations that serve various functions beyond the active pharmaceutical ingredient (API). These substances play crucial roles in enhancing the stability, bioavailability, manufacturability, and patient acceptability of medicinal products. Common categories of pharmaceutical aids include diluents, binders, disintegrants, lubricants, glidants, and preservatives. Each type of excipient contributes uniquely to the overall performance of the dosage form. For instance, diluents provide bulk to small-dose drugs, while binders ensure tablet cohesion. Disintegrants facilitate the break-up of solid dosage forms in the gastrointestinal tract, enhancing drug release. The selection of appropriate pharmaceutical aids is a critical aspect of formulation development, requiring consideration of drug-excipient compatibility, stability, and regulatory compliance. Recent advancements in excipient technology have led to the development of multifunctional excipients and those derived from natural sources, addressing the growing demand for improved drug delivery systems and environmentally friendly options.

Keywords: *Excipients, Formulation, Drug delivery, Stability, Bioavailability, Multifunctional aids*

Learning Objectives

After completion of the chapter, the student should be able to:

- Define pharmaceutical aids and their role in drug formulation.
- Classify different types of pharmaceutical aids based on their functions.
- Describe the properties and applications of common excipients.
- Explain the importance of selecting appropriate pharmaceutical aids for specific dosage forms.
- Discuss the regulatory considerations for pharmaceutical aids.
- Analyze the impact of pharmaceutical aids on drug bioavailability and stability.
- Evaluate the safety and toxicity concerns associated with various pharmaceutical aids.

Organoleptic agents promote appearance & palatability of the pharmaceutical dosage form & contribute to the acceptance of the pharmaceutical product. Coloring, flavoring and sweetening agents are grouped together as organoleptic agents.

COLORING AGENTS

Coloring agents play a crucial role that extends far beyond mere aesthetics. These additives serve multiple purposes in drug formulations, contributing significantly to product efficacy, safety, and patient compliance.

Functions of Coloring Agents

Coloring agents in pharmaceutical products serve several important functions. Primarily, they enhance the visual appeal of dosage forms, making medications more attractive to patients. This aesthetic improvement can have a profound impact on patient compliance, as visually pleasing medications are often perceived more positively.

Beyond aesthetics, coloring agents play a vital role in product identification and differentiation. In a clinical setting, where multiple medications may look similar, color coding becomes an essential safety measure. This is particularly crucial for potentially toxic or poisonous substances, where distinct coloration can prevent accidental misuse.

Interestingly, while coloring agents do not possess direct therapeutic effects, they can exert significant psychological influences on patients. The color of a medication can affect a patient's perception of its efficacy, potentially influencing the placebo effect and overall treatment outcomes.

Sources of Coloring Agents

Coloring agents used in pharmaceuticals originate from three primary sources: mineral, plant, and animal kingdoms. Each source offers unique properties and considerations for formulators.

Mineral Colors

Mineral-based colors are primarily utilized in externally applied preparations due to potential toxicity concerns when ingested. These inorganic compounds include ferric oxides (red and yellow variants), carbon black, lead chromate, and Prussian blue. While they offer excellent stability and intensity, their use is limited to topical formulations to ensure patient safety.

Plant-Based Colors

The plant kingdom provides a rich array of natural coloring agents, which are increasingly popular due to the growing demand for natural ingredients. Plant-derived colors include:

Flavones: This group encompasses compounds like rutin, riboflavin, hesperidin, quercetin, and beta-carotene, which impart various shades of yellow to formulations.

Table: Comparison of Different Color Sources

Source	Advantages	Disadvantages	Common Uses
Mineral	Stable, intense colors	Limited to external use, potential toxicity	Topical preparations, external products
Plant-based	Natural origin, perceived as safer	Variable stability, batch consistency issues	Wide range of oral and topical products
Animal-sourced	Unique colors, historical significance	Ethical concerns, potential allergens	Limited use, specialty products
Synthetic	Consistent, stable, wide color range	Regulatory scrutiny, consumer perception	Majority of pharmaceutical products

Saffron and Alizarin: These natural dyes produce

reddish-yellow hues, adding warmth to pharmaceutical preparations.

Other plant pigments: Anthocyanins, chlorophyll, and carotenoids offer a spectrum of colors from reds and purples to greens and oranges.

Plant-based colors often appeal to consumers seeking natural products. However, formulators must consider potential stability issues and batch-to-batch variability when working with these natural pigments.

Animal-Sourced Colors

Although less common in modern formulations due to ethical considerations and potential allergenicity, some colors of animal origin still find specialized uses:

Tyrian blue: Extracted from the glands of certain snail species, this historically significant dye produces a deep blue color.

Cochineal: Derived from the insect Coccus cacti, this dye yields a bright red color due to its carminic acid content.

Synthetic Colors

The advent of synthetic colors revolutionized pharmaceutical coloring, offering improved consistency, stability, and a broader color palette. The U.S. Food and Drug Administration (FDA) categorizes synthetic colors into three groups:

a. Colors permitted for Food, Drugs & Cosmetics (FD&C)

b. Colors permitted for Drugs & Cosmetics (D&C)

c. Colors permitted for externally applied Drugs & Cosmetics (external D&C)

These classifications ensure appropriate use and safety across different product types.

Synthetic colors are further divided into two main categories:

Soluble Dyes

Soluble dyes, derived from petrochemicals, exhibit color by transmitted light and are water-soluble. This group includes coal tar colors such as naphthol blue black, brilliant blue, resorcin brown, sunset yellow, and tartrazine. Their water solubility makes them ideal for liquid formulations, offering vibrant and consistent coloration.

Lake Pigments

Lake pigments represent an important class of colorants, especially for oil-based formulations. These pigments are created by adsorbing metal salts of dyes onto a base, typically alumina hydrate. Their insolubility in water makes them the coloring agent of choice for oils, fats, and lipid formulations.

It's worth noting that only aluminum lake pigments are permitted for use in FDA-approved colors, ensuring a standardized approach to formulation and safety.

FLAVORING AGENTS

Flavoring agents are important components in pharmaceutical formulations, contributing to patient compliance and treatment efficacy. These agents serve to enhance the palatability of medications, particularly for pediatric and geriatric populations. Flavoring agents consist of aroma molecules combined with a carrier substance. Their primary function is to improve the taste of pharmaceutical products, either by providing a pleasant flavor or by masking unpleasant tastes common in many active pharmaceutical ingredients. Taste improvement is essential for ensuring patient adherence to medication regimens.

Classification of Flavoring Agents

Flavoring agents in pharmaceuticals are classified into three main categories:

1. Natural Flavors (N)
2. Artificial Flavors (A)
3. Natural and Artificial Flavors (N&A)

Each category has distinct characteristics, advantages, and challenges in pharmaceutical applications.

1. Natural Flavors (N)

Natural flavors are derived from plant or animal sources through processes such as distillation, extrusion, or solvent extraction. These flavors are valued for their authenticity and consumer appeal.

Common natural flavoring agents in pharmaceuticals include:

- Citrus oils (e.g., lemon, orange)
- Anise (Pimpinella anisum)
- Cardamom (Elettaria cardamomum)
- Wild Cherry (Prunus serotina)
- Peppermint (Mentha piperita)

Natural flavors have limitations, primarily their inherent instability, which can lead to variations in flavor intensity and quality over time. This instability can be problematic in pharmaceutical formulations where consistency is crucial.

2. Artificial Flavors (A)

Artificial flavors are synthesized aroma chemicals designed to mimic natural flavors. These flavors offer several advantages in pharmaceutical applications:

- Enhanced stability
- Greater consistency in flavor profile
- Less susceptibility to raw material variations

Historically, pharmaceutical flavors often included

volatile oils like anise, clove, fennel, and wintergreen, or their isolated components such as menthol, thymol, and camphor. Modern artificial flavors have expanded this range, offering a wide variety of taste profiles.

An innovative approach in flavor technology is the production of spray-dried or adsorbed powder flavors. These are created by emulsifying naturally occurring volatile oils using acacia dextrin, resulting in a stable, easily incorporated flavoring agent.

3. Natural and Artificial Flavors (N&A)

This category combines natural and artificial flavors to achieve a balance of authenticity, stability, and flavor fullness. This approach often results in superior flavor profiles that can effectively mask unpleasant tastes while maintaining a degree of naturalness.

Flavor Enhancers and Potentiators

In addition to primary flavoring agents, pharmaceutical formulators often use flavor enhancers and potentiators. These substances amplify or modify existing flavors, contributing to a more rounded taste experience. Common flavor enhancers include:

- Sugars
- Carboxylic acids (e.g., citric acid, malic acid, tartaric acid)
- Common salt (NaCl)
- Amino acids and their derivatives (e.g., monosodium glutamate - MSG)
- Spices (e.g., various peppers)
- Monoammonium glycyrrhizinate

Flavor Profiles and Associated Tastes

Understanding the association between specific flavors and taste perceptions is important for effective flavor formulation. Some common associations include:

- Alkaline taste: Mint, chocolate, vanilla, custard

- Acidic taste: Lemon, orange, anise, licorice, raspberry, cherry, strawberry
- Bitter taste: Anise, mint, fennel, chocolate, cherry
- Metallic taste: Grape, lemon, burgundy
- Salty taste: Citrus, raspberry, fruity, melon
- Sweet taste: Fruity, vanilla, honey

Color Associations

Flavors often have color associations that can influence patient perception and acceptance of a medication. Some common flavor-color associations include:

- Pink to red: Cherry, raspberry, strawberry, apple, rose
- Brown: Chocolate, honey, walnut, caramel
- Yellow to orange: Lemon, lime, orange, custard, cherry
- Green: Banana, mint
- White to off-white: Vanilla, mint, spearmint, jasmine, banana
- Violet to purple: Violet, grape, licorice
- Blue: Blueberry, mixed fruit, plum

SWEETENING AGENTS

Taste is again a chemical sense and its appreciation results from the contact between the taste possessing materials and the **9000 taste buds in the oral cavity.**

Four primary tastes SWEET, BITTER, SOUR, SALINE are recognized and all the other tastes are considered to be admixtures of one or more fundamental tastes in varying degrees.

Sweeteners are often classied as either **caloric or noncaloric.** Non-caloric sweetening agents are preferred for diabetic patients,

Table: Examples of sweetening agents

Sweetening Agents Category	**Examples**
Caloric (contraindicated in Diabetic patients)	Sucrose/tablesugar Fructose D-Glucose
Non-caloric (Sugar free sweeteners)	Saccharine (500 times sweeter than sucrose; unpleasant aftertaste) Aspartame (200 times sweeter than sucrose; unstable in solution) Acesulfame-K (200 times sweeter than sucrose; Heat stable) Cyclamate/Na. cyclamate (30 times sweeter than sucrose) Sorbitol (polyols) Sucralose (600 times sweeter than sucrose)

The commonly used sweeteners in the pharmaceutical industry are sucrose (sugar), glucose, fructose, sorbitol, and glycerin. Mannitol is used in manufacturing of chewable tablet. It is less hygroscopic & has negative heat of solution.

Sugar-free sweeteners

In pharmaceutical formulations, sugar-free sweeteners play a crucial role in improving the palatability of medications while avoiding the potential drawbacks associated with sugar. These sweeteners are particularly important in formulations for diabetic patients and in products where sugar-induced dental caries is a concern. The following are the main categories of sugar-free sweeteners used in pharmaceutical preparations:

Sugars

- **Sugars** such as cane sugar, glucose with or without complimentary compounds like sorbitol, glycerin etc. have been used as sweetening agents from the very beginning.
- Sugar coating was an ancient technique and **simple syrup** has been used as vehicle for many oral preparations. Sugar often comprise of appreciable portions of solid dosage forms such as tablets.
- Cane sugar is stable between pH 4-8 and is generally used along with glycerin or sorbitol which reduces its tendency to get crystallized. Liquid glucose, prepared by partial hydrolysis of starch is also very suitable for sweetening of liquid preparations.
- Chief drawback with all sugars is their liability to microbial growths.
- Sugars such as **lactose and maltose**, have very limited sweetening power and as such the same are required to be used in large amounts.
- **Sucrose,** a low molecular weight carbohydrate, has been traditionally used as sweetening agent because of several advantages associated with it: very soluble in water, stable over a pH range of 4 to 8, increases viscosity which impart a product a pleasant texture in the mouth.
- Sucrose: Can not use in diabetic patients
- Polyhydric alcohols: sorbitol, mannitol, and to some extent glycerine have sweetening properties and **can be used** in preparations **for diabetic patients**

Artificial sweeteners

Artificial sweeteners are used in very small amounts of these substances can make formulations appreciably sweet. Artificial sweeteners includes

1. **Saccharin**
2. **Aspartame**
3. **cyclamates**
4. **Acesulphame-K**
5. **Acesulphame**

Saccharin

- Saccharin is marketed as saccharin sodium in which the hydrogen in –NH group is replaced by Na and which in the crystalline form also has two molecules of water o crystallization. Sodium saccharine can be easily prepared by dissolving saccharin in equimolecular quantities of aqueous sodium hydroxide solution followed by crystallization. Sodium saccharin is nearly 200 times more soluble in water in comparison to saccharin.
- **Saccharin is reputed to be nearly 450-500 times sweeter**
- **Saccharin does not undergo metabolism and its potential for causing cancer is determining factor for its use(carcinogen** due to cyclohexylamine formation, possibly by gut microbiota)
- Leaves bitter after taste

Aspartame

- 200 times sweeter than sucrose
- **Aspartame** undergoes metabolism producing phenylalanine and the phenylalanine metabolism is a problem in persons with **phenylketonuria**

Cyclamate/ Sodium cyclamate

- 30 times as sweet as sugar
- Carcinogenic potential so banned in USA
- No after taste

Sucralose

- 600 times sweeter than sucrose

Acesulphame

- approximately 200 times sweeter than sucrose

Monoammonium glycyrrhizinate

- Monoammonium glycyrrhizinate used in **liquid oral preparations**

PRESERVATIVES

Preservatives play a crucial role in maintaining the safety, efficacy, and stability of pharmaceutical and cosmetic products throughout their shelf life. These substances are added to prevent microbial growth, which could otherwise compromise product integrity and potentially harm consumers. The use of preservatives is particularly important in multi-dose formulations, where repeated exposure to the environment and potential contaminants necessitates ongoing protection against microbial proliferation.

Microbial Organisms in Pharmaceutical and Cosmetic Products

The microbial organisms associated with pharmaceutical and cosmetic products are typically categorized into three groups: harmful organisms, objectionable organisms, and opportunistic organisms. Each category presents different levels of risk and requires specific considerations in product formulation and preservation strategies.

Harmful Organisms

Harmful organisms are those directly responsible for causing human disease or infection. Their presence in pharmaceutical or cosmetic products poses an immediate and significant risk to consumer health. Examples of harmful organisms include Salmonella species, Escherichia coli, Pseudomonas aeruginosa, and Staphylococcus aureus. These pathogens are known to cause a range of infections and diseases, from mild skin irritations to severe systemic infections. The presence of any of these organisms in a product is considered unacceptable, and stringent quality control measures are implemented to ensure their absence.

Objectionable Organisms

Objectionable organisms, while not always directly harmful, have the potential to cause disease, interfere with drug function, or lead to product deterioration. This category includes organisms such as Pseudomonas putida, Pseudomonas multivorans, Pseudomonas maltophilia, Proteus mirabilis, Serratia marcescens, Klebsiella species, Acinetobacter anitratus, and Candida species. The presence of these organisms can compromise product integrity or effectiveness, potentially leading to reduced therapeutic efficacy or altered product characteristics. While they may not pose an immediate health threat to all users, their presence is considered undesirable and may render a product unsuitable for use.

Opportunistic Organisms

Opportunistic pathogens represent a unique challenge in product preservation. These organisms can produce disease or infection under specific environmental conditions or in individuals with compromised immune systems. While they may not pose a significant threat to healthy individuals, they can cause serious infections in vulnerable populations such as newborns, the elderly, or immunocompromised individuals. The specific types of opportunistic organisms can vary, but often include certain species of Pseudomonas, Acinetobacter, and various fungi. The presence of these organisms in pharmaceutical or cosmetic products requires careful consideration of the intended user population and potential risks.

Preservative Use in Different Formulations

The need for preservatives varies depending on the type of formulation and its intended use. Single-use formulations or containers generally do not require preservatives, as the product is used immediately, leaving insufficient time for bacterial colonization. However, multi-dose drug products must contain preservatives to prevent bacterial growth during storage and repeated use.

Commonly used preservatives for oral preparations include p-hydroxybenzoic acid esters and salts of benzoic acid. These compounds are chosen for their adequate solubility in aqueous systems and their broad-spectrum antimicrobial activity against both fungi and bacteria.

Ideal Properties of Preservatives

To be effective and safe for use in pharmaceutical and cosmetic products, preservatives should possess several key properties:

1. Non-irritating: The preservative should not cause irritation to the skin, eyes, or other tissues it may contact.
2. Non-toxic: It must be safe for human use, even with prolonged exposure.
3. Stability: The preservative should maintain its physical and chemical stability throughout the

product's shelf life.

4. Compatibility: It should be compatible with other ingredients in the formulation, not causing any unwanted interactions or degradation.
5. Broad-spectrum activity: An ideal preservative should be effective against a wide range of microorganisms, including bacteria, fungi, and yeasts.
6. Potency: It should be effective at low concentrations to minimize potential side effects and reduce costs.
7. Persistent activity: The preservative should maintain its antimicrobial activity throughout the manufacturing process, product shelf life, and during consumer use

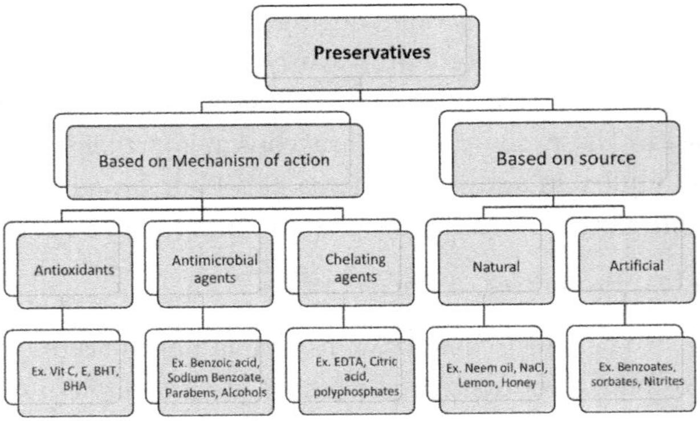

Figure 4.1: Classification of preservatives

Types of Preservatives

I. On the basis of mechanism of action

i) Antimicrobial agents

Antimicrobial agents act against microorganisms by affecting various cellular portions of microbial cells, thereby inhibiting their growth. The primary targets for these preservatives are the cell wall, cytoplasmic membrane, and cytoplasm. Antimicrobial agents used as preservatives can be classified into four major groups: acidic, neutral, mercurial, and quaternary ammonium compounds.

Acidic Antimicrobial agents are widely used in oral pharmaceuticals due to their characteristic properties. While phenols are less common in oral preparations due to their distinct odor and instability when exposed to oxygen, p-hydroxybenzoic acid esters and the salts of benzoic and sorbic acid are frequently employed. These compounds possess both antifungal and antibacterial properties and have favorable aqueous solubility. To achieve the desired antimicrobial effect, a combination of two or more esters of parahydroxybenzoic acid is often used. For instance, methyl and propyl parahydroxybenzoic acid are commonly combined in a ratio of 10 to 1, respectively.

The remaining three classes of preservatives - neutral, mercurial, and quaternary ammonium compounds - have found widespread use in ophthalmic, nasal, and parenteral preparations. These formulations often require more specialized preservatives due to their sensitive nature and specific routes of administration.

ii) Antioxidants

Antioxidants are self-reducing agents that oxidize themselves, thereby preventing the oxidation of components sensitive to oxygen. They play a crucial role in maintaining the stability and efficacy of pharmaceutical and cosmetic products that are prone to oxidative degradation. Antioxidants can be broadly categorized into three main types based on their mechanism of action.

True Antioxidants, which are typically water-insoluble, act by a chain-termination mechanism by reacting with free radicals. Examples of true antioxidants include butylated hydroxyanisole (BHA) and butylated hydroxytoluene (BHT). These compounds are particularly effective in preventing oxidation in oil-based formulations.

Reducing Agents, which are generally water-soluble, have a lower redox potential than the drug and get preferentially oxidized. A common example is ascorbic acid (Vitamin C). It's important to note that reducing agents can be consumed during the shelf-life of the product, which may necessitate careful formulation to ensure continued efficacy throughout the product's lifespan.

Antioxidant Synergists, also known as chelating agents, enhance the effect of antioxidants. These compounds, such as ethylenediamine tetraacetic acid (EDTA), citric acid, and tartaric acid, work by forming complexes with trace amounts of heavy metal ions, thereby inactivating their catalytic activity in the oxidation of medicaments. The use of antioxidant synergists can significantly improve the overall antioxidant efficacy of a formulation.

iii) Chelating Agents

Chelating agents are compounds that form complexes with metal ions, effectively removing them from solution. In the context of preservatives, chelating agents are particularly valuable for enhancing the effectiveness of antioxidants. By forming complexes with trace amounts of heavy metal ions, chelating agents inactivate the catalytic activity of these ions in the oxidation of medicaments. This synergistic effect can significantly improve the overall stability and shelf-life of pharmaceutical and cosmetic products.

Common examples of chelating agents used in pharmaceutical formulations include ethylenediamine tetraacetic acid (EDTA) derivatives and salts, dihydroxyethyl glycine, citric acid, and tartaric acid. These compounds are often used in conjunction with other preservatives to create a more robust preservation system, particularly in products that are sensitive to oxidation or metal-catalyzed degradation.

II. On the basis of Source

i) Natural Preservatives

Natural preservatives are substances obtained from natural sources such as plants, minerals, or animals. These preservatives have gained increasing popularity in recent years due to consumer preferences for "natural" products and concerns about synthetic chemicals. Examples of natural preservatives include neem oil, which has antimicrobial properties; salt (sodium chloride), which has been used for centuries to preserve food and can also be used in certain pharmaceutical formulations; lemon, which contains natural acids that can inhibit microbial growth; and honey, which has both antimicrobial and antioxidant properties.

While natural preservatives can be effective in certain applications, they may have limitations in terms of broad-spectrum antimicrobial activity, stability, or compatibility with other ingredients. Therefore, their use often requires careful formulation and testing to ensure adequate preservation of the product.

ii) Artificial Preservatives

Artificial preservatives are synthetic compounds created through chemical synthesis to combat various microorganisms at small concentrations. These preservatives have been extensively studied and are widely used in the pharmaceutical and cosmetic industries due to their consistent performance, broad-spectrum activity, and well-understood safety profiles. Examples of artificial preservatives include benzoates, sodium benzoate, sorbates, propionates, and nitrites.

Artificial preservatives offer several advantages, including predictable efficacy, stability across a wide range of formulations, and the ability to provide preservation at very low concentrations. However, there has been increasing scrutiny of certain artificial preservatives due to concerns about potential long-term health effects or environmental impact.

Summary

Pharmaceutical aids, also known as excipients, are essential components in drug formulations that serve a wide array of functions beyond merely bulking up the active ingredient. These inert substances play crucial roles in enhancing the stability, bioavailability, and manufacturability of pharmaceutical products. Diluents, such as lactose and microcrystalline cellulose, provide bulk and improve flow properties in solid dosage forms. Binders, including povidone and starch, help hold particles together in tablets and granules. Disintegrants, like croscarmellose sodium and sodium starch glycolate, facilitate the break-up of solid dosage forms in the gastrointestinal tract, promoting drug release. Lubricants, such as magnesium stearate, reduce friction during tablet compression and ejection. Glidants, like colloidal silicon dioxide, improve powder flow during manufacturing. Preservatives, including parabens and benzalkonium chloride, prevent microbial growth in liquid and semi-solid formulations. Antioxidants, such as butylated hydroxyanisole (BHA) and ascorbic acid, protect drugs susceptible to oxidation. Solubilizers and surfactants, like polysorbates and sodium lauryl sulfate, enhance the dissolution of poorly water-soluble drugs. Emulsifying agents, including lecithin and poloxamers, stabilize emulsions and suspensions. pH adjusters and buffers maintain the optimal pH for drug stability and efficacy. Tonicity agents, such as sodium chloride and dextrose, ensure that parenteral formulations are isotonic with body fluids. Flavoring agents and sweeteners improve the palatability of oral liquid formulations, especially important in pediatric medicines. Coloring agents, both natural and synthetic, aid in product identification and aesthetic appeal. The selection of appropriate pharmaceutical aids involves careful consideration of their physicochemical properties, compatibility with the active ingredient, and regulatory status. Quality control of excipients is rigorous, with specifications outlined in pharmacopoeias and regulatory guidelines to ensure consistency and safety in pharmaceutical formulations.

Multiple Choice Questions

1. Which of the following is NOT considered a pharmaceutical aid?
   a) Excipient
   b) Active pharmaceutical ingredient
   c) Preservative
   d) Lubricant
2. What is the primary function of a lubricant in tablet formulation?
   a) Reduce friction during tableting
   b) Increase tablet hardness
   c) Enhance drug dissolution
   d) Prevent microbial growth

3. Which of the following is commonly used as a suspending agent?
   a) Magnesium stearate
   b) Xanthan gum
   c) Lactose
   d) Aspartame
4. What is the main purpose of using a disintegrant in tablet formulation?
   a) Increase tablet hardness
   b) Enhance flavor
   c) Promote tablet break-up in the gastrointestinal tract
   d) Prevent moisture absorption
5. Which of the following is an example of a preservative?
   a) Methylparaben
   b) Starch
   c) Talc
   d) Sucrose
6. What is the primary function of an antioxidant in pharmaceutical formulations?
   a) Enhance drug absorption
   b) Prevent oxidation of ingredients
   c) Increase viscosity
   d) Mask bitter taste
7. Which of the following is commonly used as a sweetening agent in liquid formulations?
   a) Sodium lauryl sulfate
   b) Sorbitol
   c) Carboxymethylcellulose
   d) Propylene glycol
8. What is the main purpose of using a binder in tablet formulation?
   a) Enhance drug stability
   b) Increase tablet hardness and cohesiveness

c) Promote disintegration
d) Reduce friction during tableting

9. Which of the following is an example of a surfactant?
a) Polysorbate 80
b) Microcrystalline cellulose
c) Glycerin
d) Calcium phosphate

10. What is the primary function of a colorant in pharmaceutical formulations?
a) Enhance drug stability
b) Improve taste
c) Provide visual identification
d) Increase bioavailability

11. Which of the following is commonly used as a film-forming agent in tablet coating?
a) Hydroxypropyl methylcellulose
b) Magnesium stearate
c) Lactose
d) Sodium starch glycolate

12. What is the main purpose of using a plasticizer in pharmaceutical formulations?
a) Increase brittleness
b) Enhance flexibility and reduce brittleness
c) Promote disintegration
d) Prevent microbial growth

13. Which of the following is an example of a pH adjuster?
a) Citric acid
b) Povidone
c) Stearic acid
d) Mannitol

14. What is the primary function of a chelating agent in pharmaceutical formulations?
a) Enhance drug absorption

b) Prevent oxidation
c) Bind metal ions to improve stability
d) Increase viscosity

15. Which of the following is commonly used as an emulsifying agent?
a) Lecithin
b) Talc
c) Lactose
d) Calcium carbonate

16. What is the main purpose of using a glidant in tablet formulation?
a) Enhance drug dissolution
b) Improve powder flow
c) Increase tablet hardness
d) Prevent microbial growth

17. Which of the following is an example of a bulking agent in freeze-dried products?
a) Mannitol
b) Benzyl alcohol
c) Sodium lauryl sulfate
d) Propylparaben

18. What is the primary function of a wetting agent in pharmaceutical formulations?
a) Increase drug solubility
b) Enhance tablet hardness
c) Prevent microbial growth
d) Mask bitter taste

19. Which of the following is commonly used as a tablet diluent?
a) Microcrystalline cellulose
b) Methylcellulose
c) Propylene glycol
d) Sodium benzoate

20. What is the main purpose of using an adsorbent in pharmaceutical formulations?

a) Enhance drug stability
b) Improve taste
c) Absorb excess moisture or oil
d) Increase bioavailability.

List of Important Questions

1. What are pharmaceutical aids, and why are they important in drug formulation?
2. How are pharmaceutical aids classified based on their functions?
3. What are the key properties of diluents, and how do they affect tablet formulation?
4. Describe the role of binders in solid dosage form manufacturing.
5. How do disintegrants contribute to the performance of tablets and capsules?
6. What are the different types of lubricants used in pharmaceutical formulations, and how do they work?
7. Explain the importance of glidants in improving powder flow properties.
8. How do preservatives contribute to the stability of liquid pharmaceutical formulations?
9. What are antioxidants, and why are they used in pharmaceutical formulations?
10. Describe the role of emulsifying agents in pharmaceutical emulsions.
11. How do suspending agents improve the stability of pharmaceutical suspensions?
12. What are the key considerations in selecting sweeteners for oral liquid formulations?
13. How do coloring agents impact patient acceptance and product identification?
14. Explain the role of pH adjusters in pharmaceutical formulations.
15. What are the regulatory considerations for pharmaceutical aids in different countries?

Bibliography

1. Rowe RC, Sheskey PJ, Quinn ME, editors. Handbook of pharmaceutical excipients. 6th ed. London: Pharmaceutical Press; 2009.
2. Augsburger LL, Hoag SW, editors. Pharmaceutical dosage forms: tablets. 3rd ed. New York: Informa Healthcare; 2008.
3. Allen LV, Ansel HC. Ansel's pharmaceutical dosage forms and drug delivery systems. 10th ed. Philadelphia: Lippincott Williams & Wilkins; 2014.
4. Aulton ME, Taylor KMG, editors. Aulton's pharmaceutics: the design and manufacture of medicines. 5th ed. Edinburgh: Elsevier; 2018.
5. Niazi SK. Handbook of pharmaceutical manufacturing formulations: compressed solid products. 2nd ed. Boca Raton: CRC Press; 2016.
6. Ghosh TK, Jasti BR, editors. Theory and practice of contemporary pharmaceutics. Boca Raton: CRC Press; 2004.
7. Banker GS, Rhodes CT, editors. Modern pharmaceutics. 4th ed. New York: Marcel Dekker; 2002.
8. Lieberman HA, Lachman L, Schwartz JB, editors. Pharmaceutical dosage forms: tablets. 2nd ed. New York: Marcel Dekker; 1989.
9. Gibson M, editor. Pharmaceutical preformulation and formulation. 2nd ed. New York: Informa Healthcare; 2009.
10. Qiu Y, Chen Y, Zhang GGZ, Liu L, Porter WR, editors. Developing solid oral dosage forms: pharmaceutical theory and practice. Burlington: Academic Press; 2009.

CHAPTER 5

SIZE REDUCTION

Author

Miss Poonam Dashrath Dighe,
Assistant professor, Dept of Pharmaceutics,
Amruthvahini College of Pharmacy, Sangamner,
Ghulewadi, Maharashtra, India

Abstract

Size reduction is a fundamental unit operation in pharmaceutical manufacturing, crucial for enhancing drug dissolution, absorption, and overall therapeutic efficacy. This process involves breaking down larger particles into smaller ones, often to achieve specific particle size distributions tailored to the needs of different dosage forms. Various mechanisms of size reduction are employed, including impact, attrition, compression, and cutting. The choice of size reduction method depends on the material properties, desired particle size, and scale of operation. Common equipment used in pharmaceutical size reduction includes ball mills, hammer mills, jet mills, and roller mills, each with its unique operating principles and applications. Factors affecting size reduction efficiency include material hardness, feed rate, and equipment design. The concept of critical size in milling is explored, along with methods for controlling and optimizing the size reduction process. Understanding particle size analysis techniques is essential for quality control and ensuring the consistency of the final product. Size reduction not only impacts the physical properties of materials but also influences their chemical and biological behavior, making it a critical consideration in drug formulation and manufacturing.

Keywords: *Comminution, Particle size distribution, Milling equipment, Process optimization, Dissolution enhancement, Quality control*

Learning Objectives

After completion of the chapter, the student should be able to:

- Define size reduction and explain its importance in pharmaceutical manufacturing.
- Describe the principles and mechanisms of size reduction.
- Identify and explain the various methods of size reduction used in pharmaceuticals.
- Compare and contrast different types of size reduction equipment.
- Discuss the factors affecting the efficiency of size reduction processes.
- Explain the concept of particle size distribution and its measurement techniques.
- Analyze the impact of size reduction on drug dissolution and bioavailability.

This process of conversion of raw material to useful product comprises many steps. Some steps are required to make raw materials ready for processing. Some steps are required to bring the final product to desired form. These unique and distinctive steps are called unit operations

Properties of unit operations:

- They are physical in nature.
- They are used invariantly in all chemical industries (approximately)
- For a specific unit operation basic concept and principle behind it as same in all industries.
- But may be differ in method of application

Unit operation may also be called separation process. The separation is generally based on any specific property called driving force.

This driving force is the deviation of that property from the equilibrium. When the driving force is high i.e. deviation from equilibrium is large separation is easy. When equilibrium achieved separation stops as equilibrium is the condition in which netflow of the property across the system is zero. For example if the separation is based on concentration and the concentration of the species is same on both the side there will no movement meaning thereby no separation.

Classification of unit operations

Heat Transfer Operation: Unit operations where temperature difference is driving force.
Mass Transfer Operations: Unit operations where concentration gradient is driving force.
Fluid Flow Operations: Unit operations where momentum gradient is driving force.
Mechanical Operations: Operations based on some external mechanical force.
Some important unit operations carried in the pharmaceutical industries are:- Distillation, Drying, Evaporation, Gas Absorption & Desorption, Liquid-Liquid Extraction, Solid-Liquid Extraction (Leaching), Crystallization, Adsorption etc

Size reduction

Size reduction, also known as comminution, involves reducing larger particles into smaller ones. This fundamental process in pharmaceutical manufacturing serves multiple purposes, particularly in enhancing drug effectiveness and formulation characteristics.

Importance and Objectives

Size reduction significantly increases surface area,

leading to improved pharmaceutical performance. For instance, micronized griseofulvin shows five-fold better absorption compared to its regular form. The process also enables better powder mixing through uniform particle size distribution and improves suspension stability by reducing sedimentation rates. Many pharmaceutical dosage forms, including capsules and inhalation powders, require specific particle sizes below 60μm for optimal effectiveness.

Material Characteristics and Processing Considerations

Different materials require specific approaches to size reduction based on their properties. Hard materials like pumice pose challenges due to equipment wear, while fibrous materials such as rauwolfia require cutting mills. Friable materials like sucrose are easily processed using hammer or fluid energy mills. Special considerations apply to plastic materials, which need chilling before processing, and hygroscopic materials, which require closed equipment processing.

Environmental and Safety Factors

Processing conditions significantly impact size reduction efficiency. Moisture content should remain below 5% to prevent material agglomeration. For inflammable materials, proper safety measures including explosion-proof electrical systems are essential. Temperature control becomes crucial for thermolabile substances like vitamins and antibiotics.

Theoretical Framework

Several theories explain the relationship between energy input and size reduction outcomes. Rittinger's theory, focusing on surface area creation, applies best to fine milling of brittle materials. Bond's theory, relating

energy to crack propagation, suits rough mill sizing. Kick's theory, addressing particle deformation, works well for large particle crushing. Walker's theory provides a unified approach encompassing these various scenarios.
Equipment Selection and Applications
Size reduction equipment selection depends on desired particle size and material properties. Cutter mills handle large pieces effectively, while impact mills produce coarse powders. Combined impact and attrition mills generate fine powders, and fluid energy mills achieve very fine particle sizes suitable for specialized applications like vitamin processing.

Energy Considerations

Size reduction processes are typically energy-intensive, with less than 2% of input energy directly contributing to size reduction. The remainder dissipates through various mechanisms including particle deformation, material transport, friction, heat generation, and equipment inefficiencies. Understanding these energy considerations helps optimize process efficiency and equipment selection.

Quality Control and Product Requirements

Final product specifications often dictate size reduction parameters. Sterile products require specialized equipment and environments, while potent drugs need contamination-free processing methods. These requirements influence both equipment selection and processing conditions to ensure product quality and safety.

Hammer Mill

The hammer mill operates through impact-based size reduction, featuring a metal casing containing a central shaft with swiveling hammers. During operation, the hammers rotate at high speeds (80 cycles per second), breaking down materials against an undulating interior casing and a replaceable screen. The mill offers rapid, continuous operation and versatile processing capabilities, though it requires careful feed rate control and may generate heat that could affect sensitive materials.

Ball Mill

Ball mills utilize a horizontal rotating cylinder containing balls that create size reduction through impact and attrition. The cylinder, which may be constructed from metal, porcelain, or rubber, contains balls occupying 30-50% of its volume. Operating at the critical speed (approximately 0.5 cycles per second), the balls create a cascading effect that maximizes grinding efficiency. While effective for various materials and capable of producing fine powders, ball mills can generate noise and may introduce contamination from wear.

Cutter Mill

This equipment employs a cutting mechanism with both stationary and rotating knives. Materials enter through a top hopper and are processed between the knives until reaching the desired size to pass through a bottom screen. The cutter mill specializes in processing soft, fibrous materials, making it particularly suitable for preparing plant materials prior to extraction.

Roller Mill

Operating through compression, the roller mill consists of two horizontal cylindrical rolls. One roll is directly powered while the other rotates through friction when material passes through the nip between them. The adjustable gap between rolls controls the degree of size reduction. This mill type excels in crushing seeds and soft tissues, particularly in preparation for extraction processes.

Fluid Energy Mill

This advanced milling system uses high-pressure fluid (typically air) injected through nozzles to create particle collision and attrition within a looped pipe system. A classifier ensures only appropriately sized particles (as small as 5μm) exit as product. The fluid energy mill offers several advantages:

The absence of mechanical grinding surfaces eliminates product contamination

Built-in cooling effect from gas expansion protects thermolabile materials

Capability to use inert gases for sensitive materials

Achieves the finest particle sizes among all milling methods

Selection Considerations

When choosing milling equipment, several factors require evaluation:

Material Properties: Consider hardness, thermosensitivity, and moisture content

Required Particle Size: Match equipment capabilities to target specifications

Production Volume: Evaluate throughput requirements and continuous vs. batch operation

Product Quality Requirements: Consider contamination risks and temperature sensitivity

Operating Costs: Factor in energy consumption and maintenance requirements

.

Summary

Size reduction is a fundamental unit operation in pharmaceutical manufacturing, crucial for enhancing drug dissolution, improving content uniformity, and facilitating further processing. This process involves the breakdown of larger particles into smaller ones through the application of mechanical forces. Various mechanisms contribute to size reduction, including impact, attrition, compression, and cutting. Impact involves particle breakage due to collision with hard surfaces or other particles. Attrition results from particles rubbing against each other or machine parts. Compression causes particle fracture under pressure, while cutting involves the use of sharp edges to slice particles. The choice of size reduction method depends on the material properties, desired particle size, and subsequent processing requirements. Mills are the primary equipment used for size reduction, with several types available for different applications. Ball mills utilize rotating cylinders filled with balls that crush and grind materials. Hammer mills employ rapidly moving hammers to shatter particles against a screen. Fluid energy mills (jet mills) use high-velocity gas streams to cause particle collisions and size reduction. Roller mills crush materials between rotating rollers, while colloid mills are used for producing fine suspensions and emulsions. Factors influencing size reduction efficiency include feed rate, mill speed, grinding medium properties, and material characteristics such as hardness and friability. The energy requirements for size reduction increase significantly as particle size decreases, following relationships described by Kick's, Rittinger's, and Bond's laws. Particle size analysis techniques, including sieve analysis, microscopy, and laser diffraction, are employed to assess the effectiveness of size reduction processes. Heat generation during milling can be a concern, particularly for thermolabile substances, necessitating cooling systems in some equipment. Containment and dust control are crucial considerations, especially when handling potent or hazardous materials.

Multiple Choice Questions

1. What is the primary purpose of size reduction in pharmaceutical manufacturing?
   a) To increase particle size
   b) To decrease particle size
   c) To change particle shape
   d) To increase bulk density
2. Which of the following is NOT a method of size reduction?
   a) Milling
   b) Grinding
   c) Crystallization
   d) Crushing
3. The energy required for size reduction is inversely proportional to:
   a) The initial particle size
   b) The final particle size
   c) The square root of the new surface area produced
   d) The hardness of the material
4. Which type of mill is most suitable for wet grinding of pharmaceuticals?
   a) Ball mill
   b) Hammer mill
   c) Fluid energy mill
   d) Roller mill

5. The principle of impaction is primarily used in which type of mill?
   a) Ball mill
   b) Hammer mill
   c) Colloid mill
   d) Fluid energy mill
6. Which of the following factors does NOT affect the efficiency of a size reduction process?
   a) Feed rate
   b) Machine capacity
   c) Material hardness
   d) Operator's age
7. What is the main advantage of cryogenic grinding?
   a) Increased particle size
   b) Reduced heat generation
   c) Higher energy efficiency
   d) Faster grinding speed
8. Which type of mill is most suitable for size reduction of heat-sensitive materials?
   a) Hammer mill
   b) Ball mill
   c) Fluid energy mill
   d) Roller mill
9. The process of size reduction where particles are broken down by high-velocity collisions with each other is called:
   a) Attrition
   b) Impaction
   c) Compression
   d) Cutting
10. Which of the following is an example of an ultra-fine grinding mill?
    a) Hammer mill
    b) Roller mill

c) Colloid mill
d) Cutting mill

11. The term "critical speed" in ball milling refers to:
a) The maximum speed at which the mill can operate
b) The speed at which balls start to centrifuge
c) The minimum speed required for size reduction
d) The speed at which the mill consumes the least energy

12. Which of the following is NOT a common problem encountered during size reduction?
a) Heat generation
b) Noise pollution
c) Particle agglomeration
d) Increased solubility

13. The principle of attrition is primarily used in which type of mill?
a) Hammer mill
b) Fluid energy mill
c) Ball mill
d) Cutting mill

14. Which of the following materials is most difficult to reduce in size?
a) Crystalline substances
b) Fibrous materials
c) Elastic materials
d) Brittle materials

15. What is the primary advantage of using a fluid energy mill?
a) Low energy consumption
b) Ability to handle wet materials
c) Production of very fine particles
d) High throughput rate

16. The process of size reduction where particles are broken down by being squeezed between two

surfaces is called:
a) Attrition
b) Impaction
c) Compression
d) Cutting

17. Which of the following factors contributes to increased energy consumption during size reduction?
a) Decreased hardness of material
b) Increased initial particle size
c) Decreased final particle size
d) Increased moisture content

18. What is the main disadvantage of using a ball mill for size reduction?
a) Inability to handle hard materials
b) High noise levels
c) Long processing times
d) Inability to produce fine particles

19. Which type of mill is most suitable for size reduction of thermolabile materials?
a) Hammer mill
b) Fluid energy mill
c) Roller mill
d) Colloid mill

20. The phenomenon where further size reduction becomes difficult below a certain particle size is known as:
a) Aggregation limit
b) Grinding limit
c) Critical size
d) Comminution threshold.

List of Important Questions

1. What is size reduction, and why is it important in pharmaceutical manufacturing?
2. How does particle size affect the properties and performance of pharmaceutical products?
3. What are the main mechanisms of size reduction in pharmaceutical processing?
4. Describe the principle of operation of a ball mill.
5. How does a hammer mill work, and what are its applications in pharmaceuticals?
6. What are the advantages and disadvantages of fluid energy mills?
7. Explain the working principle of a colloid mill and its applications.
8. How does cryogenic grinding differ from conventional grinding methods?
9. What factors affect the efficiency of a size reduction process?
10. How is the energy requirement for size reduction calculated?
11. Describe the safety considerations in size reduction operations.
12. What are the challenges in size reduction of heat-sensitive materials?
13. How does wet grinding differ from dry grinding in terms of process and applications?
14. Explain the concept of critical speed in ball milling.
15. What are the latest innovations in size reduction technology for pharmaceuticals?

Bibliography

1. Staniforth J. Powder flow. In: Aulton ME, editor. Pharmaceutics: the science of dosage form design. 2nd ed. Edinburgh: Churchill Livingstone; 2002. p. 197-210.
2. Allen T. Particle size measurement. 5th ed. London: Chapman & Hall; 1997.
3. Shekunov BY, Chattopadhyay P, Tong HHY, Chow AHL. Particle size analysis in pharmaceutics: principles, methods and applications. Pharm Res. 2007;24(2):203-27.
4. Parrott EL. Milling of pharmaceutical solids. J Pharm Sci. 1974;63(6):813-29.
5. Lachman L, Lieberman HA, Kanig JL. The theory and practice of industrial pharmacy. 3rd ed. Philadelphia: Lea & Febiger; 1986.
6. Aulton ME, Taylor KMG, editors. Aulton's pharmaceutics: the design and manufacture of medicines. 5th ed. Edinburgh: Elsevier; 2018.
7. Rhodes MJ. Introduction to particle technology. 2nd ed. Chichester: John Wiley & Sons; 2008.
8. Kwan CC, Chen YQ, Ding YL, Papadopoulos DG, Bentham AC, Ghadiri M. Development of a novel approach towards predicting the milling behaviour of pharmaceutical powders. Eur J Pharm Sci. 2004;23(4-5):327-36.
9. Otsuka M, Yamane I. Prediction of tablet properties based on near infrared spectra of raw mixed powders by chemometrics: scale-up factor of blending and tableting processes. J Pharm Sci. 2009;98(11):4296-305.
10. Bauer-Brandl A, Becker D. Milling. In: Swarbrick J, editor. Encyclopedia of pharmaceutical technology. 3rd ed. NY: Informa Healthcare; 2007. p. 2328-38.

CHAPTER 6

SIZE SEPARATION

Author

Mr. Gaurav Pratap Singh,
Assistant Professor, Dr. K N Modi Institute of Pharmaceutical Education & Research, Modinagar, Uttar Pradesh, India

Abstract

Size separation is a crucial process in pharmaceutical manufacturing that involves the classification of particles based on their size. This operation is essential for achieving uniform particle size distributions, which directly impact drug dissolution, bioavailability, and manufacturing efficiency. Various methods of size separation are employed, including sieving, elutriation, and sedimentation. Sieving, the most common technique, uses a series of mesh screens to separate particles of different sizes. The principles of sieve analysis and the importance of selecting appropriate sieve sizes are discussed. Factors affecting sieving efficiency, such as particle shape, moisture content, and sieving time, are examined. Air classification and cyclone separators are explored as alternatives for fine powder separation. The concept of particle size distribution and its measurement using various techniques, including laser diffraction and image analysis, is introduced. Size separation plays a critical role in quality control, ensuring batch-to-batch consistency and meeting regulatory requirements for particle size specifications.

Keywords: *Sieving, Particle classification, Size distribution, Powder technology, Quality control, Batch uniformity*

Learning Objectives

After completion of the chapter, the student should be able to:

- Define size separation and its significance in pharmaceutical processing.
- Explain the principles of various size separation techniques.
- Describe different types of sieves and sieving equipment used in pharmaceuticals.
- Discuss the factors affecting the efficiency of size separation processes.
- Explain the concept of particle size analysis and its importance.
- Compare and contrast different methods of particle size measurement.
- Analyze the applications of size separation in various pharmaceutical operations.

SIZE SEPARATION

Size separation (or classification) is a process in which particles of desired size are separated from other fractions.

Classification of powders according to IP

During the process of size reduction, it is not possible to obtain the particle of uniform size. Hence special technique is used to **separate particles of a specified size**, which is known as the process of size separation. Size separation is also known as sieving, sifting, screening. This technique is based on physical differences b/w the particles such as size, shape and density

When the fineness of the powder is described by

means of a number, it is intended that all the particles of the powder shall pass through a sieve of which the nominal mesh aperture, in μm , is equal to that number.

Official Standard for Powder: IP (Indian Pharmacopoeia). Coarse or fineness of powder is expressed by Reference to the nominal mesh aperture size of the sieve through which powder is able to pass.

Table: Indian pharmacopoeia- 5 grade of powder

S. No.	**Grade of powder**	**All particles must pass through Sieve No. /Nominal mesh aperture**	**Sieve through which 40% of the particles pass/ Nominal mesh aperture**
1	Coarse powder	10 /(1700 μm)	44 /(355 μm)
2	Moderately coarse powder	22 /(710 μm)	60/ (250 μm)
3	Moderately fine powder	44/(355 μm)	85/(180 **μm**)
4	Fine powder	85/(180 μm)	Not specified
5	Very fine powder	120/(125 μm)	Not specified

Official Grade of powder as per Indian Pharmacopoeia/IP

A) Coarse Powder:

- All the particles of which pass through a sieve with nominal mesh aperture of 1.70 mm/1700 μm (**Sieve No. 10**) and not more than 40% pass through nominal mesh aperture of 355 μm (**Sieve No. 44**) is called a **Coarse Powder**.

B) Moderately Coarse Powder:

- All the particles of which pass through a sieve with nominal mesh aperture of 710 μm (**Sieve No. 22**) and not more than 40% pass through nominal mesh aperture of 250 μm (**Sieve No. 60**) is called a **Moderately Coarse Powder.**

C) Moderately Fine Powder:

- All the particles of which pass through a sieve with nominal mesh aperture of 355 μm (**Sieve No. 44**) and not more than 40% pass through nominal mesh aperture of 180 μm (**Sieve No. 85**) is called a **Moderately Fine Powder.**

D) Fine Powder:

- All the particles of which pass through a sieve with nominal mesh aperture of 180 μm (**Sieve No. 85**) is called a **Fine Powder.**

E) Very Fine Powder:

- All the particles of which pass through a sieve with nominal mesh aperture of 125 μm (**Sieve No. 120**) is called a **Fine Powder.**
- **Note:**
  - For Fine & Very fine grade of powder: IP has prescribed only the upper limit (Fine & Very fine)
  - Fineness of powder is described by means of Number: it indicates that all particles of powder shall pass through that sieve number (respective nominal mesh aperture in μm).

F) Microfine powder

A powder of which not less than 90 percent by weight of the particles pass through a sieve with a nominal mesh aperture of 45 μm.

G) Superfine powder

A powder of which not less than 90 percent by a number of the particles are less than 10 μm in size.

Cyclone separator

Principle

Cyclone separator is a type of sedimentation technique that works on the principle of centrifugal force rather than gravitational force. Thus, based on the fluid velocity, a cyclone enables the separation of all the particles or only the coarse particles can be removed, leaving behind the particles which are then carried away by the fluid.

Construction

Comprising a cylindrical vessel with a conical base, the cyclone separator is designed to optimize its functionality. The upper section of the vessel is equipped with a tangential inlet and a fluid outlet, while the base is fitted with a solid outlet for particle discharge.

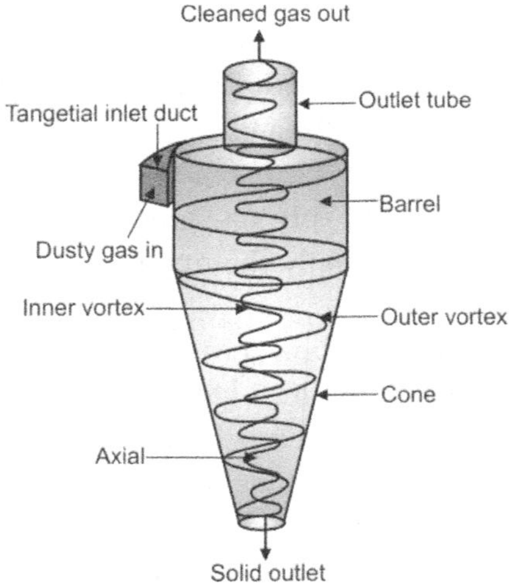

Figure: Cyclone Separator

Working

To initiate the process, a gas suspension carrying solid particles, typically air, is introduced into the vessel with a tangential entry at an exceptionally high velocity, thereby creating a rotational motion within the system. The fluid is subsequently extracted from a central outlet located at the top. As the gas circulates within the cyclone separator, the centrifugal force comes into play, exerting its influence on the particles. This force propels the solids towards the walls, ultimately leading them to descend and collect at the conical base, ready for expulsion through the solids outlet.

Applications

The applications of cyclone separators extend to the separation of solid suspensions in gas, particularly air. Additionally, these separators can also be utilized for liquid suspensions containing solid particles. By harnessing the power of centrifugal force, cyclone separators provide an effective means of achieving particle separation and enhancing the efficiency of various processes.

In pharmaceuticals, it employs cyclones to segregate fine particles from larger granules. These cyclones play an important role in tablet compression by extracting excess powder, ensuring it is removed prior to reaching the central extraction system.

Advantages:

- It is Highly Efficient
- Cost-Effectiveness
- Compact and Space-Saving

Disadvantages:

- Cyclone separators require adequate space for installation due to their design.
- Required more energy input.

- Required a Large amount of air to be introduced.

Cyclone Separator Variants

The cyclone separator, a versatile apparatus, finds utility not only in gas-solid separation but also in the separation of solid particles suspended in a liquid medium. This variant, known as a wet or liquid cyclone, capitalizes on the contrasting densities of the solid and liquid particles involved. Notably, when dealing with a liquid suspension, the task becomes more intricate due to the heightened viscosity of water in comparison to air.

To achieve effective separation in such cases, a greater centrifugal force must be exerted. One method to amplify this force involves reducing the diameter of the vessel, thereby intensifying the effects of centrifugation. As the cyclone separator operates, coarse particles, propelled outward by the formidable centrifugal force, the journey toward the vessel walls and eventually gather at its base. Concurrently, the lighter particles, alongside the liquid medium, make their escape through the outlet positioned atop the vessel. This interplay of forces and dynamics showcases the efficient functionality of the cyclone separator in the context of liquid-solid particle separation.

SIEVE ANALYSIS

Equivalent Diameter

In sieve analysis, the sieve diameter (ds) represents a critical measurement parameter that defines how particles interact with the mesh openings. The sieve diameter corresponds to the dimension of a particle that can pass through a square aperture of length x. This concept is fundamental to understanding particle size distribution, though it's important to note that the actual particle shape can influence passage through the sieve apertures.

Range of Analysis

The International Standards Organization (ISO) has established standardized parameters for sieve analysis, setting the lower limit at 45 micrometers. While powders are conventionally defined as particles with maximum diameters of 1000 micrometers, practical applications of sieve analysis extend far beyond these bounds. Modern sieving equipment can effectively analyze particles ranging from as small as 5 micrometers to as large as 125000 micrometers, making it an incredibly versatile analytical technique for various industrial and pharmaceutical applications.

Sample Preparation

Sample preparation plays a crucial role in achieving accurate and reproducible results. Most commonly, powders are analyzed in their dry state, as this provides the most straightforward and reliable results. However, the technique's versatility allows for the analysis of powders suspended in liquid media, though this requires special considerations and modified procedures to ensure accurate measurements.

Principle of Measurement with Sieve

The fundamental principle of sieve analysis involves the systematic separation of particles using a series of mesh screens with progressively smaller apertures. These screens, typically constructed from brass or stainless steel, create physical barriers that separate particles based on size. The sieves are arranged in a vertical stack, often called a 'nest' or 'stack,' with the largest apertures at the top and smallest at the bottom. This arrangement facilitates the gradual separation of particles as they move downward through the stack.

A typical analysis employs 6 to 8 sieves, with aperture sizes following a geometric progression based on either a factor of 2 or √2 between adjacent sieves. The process begins by placing a known weight (W0) of the sample on the topmost sieve. After securing the stack, it undergoes controlled agitation for a predetermined period. Following the shaking period, each sieve is carefully separated, and the retained material is weighed and recorded. This systematic approach allows for the creation of a detailed particle size distribution profile.

Standards of Sieves

The effectiveness and reliability of sieve analysis depend heavily on standardized sieve construction and specifications. Wire-mesh sieves must be manufactured using wire of uniform, circular cross-section. Each sieve carries specific identifiers and characteristics that must be clearly stated:

The sieve number indicates the mesh density, specifically the number of openings within a 25.4mm (1-inch) length in both directions. The nominal aperture size defines the distance between wires, essentially representing the side length of the square openings. This measurement is crucial as it determines the maximum spherical particle size that can pass through, though it's worth noting that non-spherical particles may pass through differently depending on their orientation.

The wire diameter plays a dual role in sieve construction. Beyond forming the mesh structure, it must provide sufficient strength to maintain the aperture dimensions during use. The wire diameter is typically specified using the Standard Wire Gauge system, ensuring consistency across different manufacturers and applications.

Screen area represents another critical parameter in sieve design. The approximate screen area, expressed as a percentage, indicates the ratio of open area to total sieve area. This value typically falls between 35% and 45% of the total area, with higher percentages generally preferred for improved efficiency. The relationship between wire diameter and aperture size directly influences this parameter.

Aperture tolerance average acknowledges the practical limitations in manufacturing perfectly uniform sieves. This tolerance, expressed as a percentage, defines acceptable variations in aperture dimensions. Notably, finer meshes typically require larger tolerance ranges due to the increased complexity in maintaining precise dimensions with finer wires.

The Tyler Standard Screen Scale provides a widely recognized reference system for sieve specifications, offering standardized relationships between mesh numbers, aperture sizes, and wire diameters. This standardization ensures consistency and reproducibility in particle size analysis across different laboratories and applications.

Summary

Size separation is a critical unit operation in pharmaceutical manufacturing, employed to classify particles based on their dimensions and ensure uniformity in drug formulations. This process is essential for achieving desired product specifications, improving flow properties, and enhancing the dissolution characteristics of pharmaceutical materials. Various methods of size separation are utilized, each suited to different particle size ranges and material properties. Sieving, one of the most common techniques, involves passing particles through a series of screens with progressively smaller apertures. Mechanical sieving employs vibration or rotation to facilitate particle passage, while air jet sieving uses upward air currents to deagglomerate particles. Elutriation separates particles based on their terminal settling velocity in a fluid stream, typically air or water. Cyclone separators utilize centrifugal force to separate particles of different sizes and densities. Hydrocyclones apply similar principles but use water as the separation medium. Centrifugal sedimentation techniques, including disc centrifuges and tubular bowl centrifuges, are employed for fine particle separation, particularly in liquid suspensions. Filtration methods, ranging from simple strainers to advanced membrane filtration systems, separate particles based on size exclusion principles. The selection of an appropriate size separation method depends on factors such as particle size range, material properties, desired throughput, and the presence of agglomerates. Particle size analysis techniques, including laser diffraction, dynamic light scattering, and image analysis, are used to assess the effectiveness of separation processes. The efficiency of size separation is influenced by various factors, including particle shape, density, surface properties, and the presence of electrostatic charges. Challenges in size separation include dealing with near-size particles, preventing re-agglomeration, and maintaining separation efficiency over time. In pharmaceutical manufacturing, size separation is often integrated with other unit operations, such as milling and granulation, to achieve precise particle size distributions critical for drug product performance and quality.

Multiple Choice Questions

1. Which of the following is NOT a method of size separation?
   a) Sieving
   b) Elutriation
   c) Sedimentation
   d) Crystallization
2. The process of separating particles based on their terminal falling velocity in a fluid is called:
   a) Sieving
   b) Elutriation
   c) Filtration
   d) Cyclone separation
3. Which of the following factors does NOT affect the efficiency of a sieving process?
   a) Mesh size
   b) Particle shape
   c) Sieve motion
   d) Particle color
4. The term "mesh number" in sieving refers to:
   a) The number of wires per linear inch of the sieve
   b) The total number of openings in the sieve
   c) The thickness of the wire used in the sieve
   d) The total surface area of the sieve

5. Which of the following size separation techniques is most suitable for separating very fine particles?
   a) Standard sieving
   b) Air classification
   c) Gravitational sedimentation
   d) Magnetic separation
6. The principle of centrifugal force is used in which of the following size separation techniques?
   a) Sieving
   b) Elutriation
   c) Cyclone separation
   d) Filtration
7. Which of the following is an advantage of air classification over sieving?
   a) Lower energy consumption
   b) Ability to handle wet materials
   c) More precise size separation
   d) Simpler equipment design
8. The process of separating particles based on their ability to pass through a porous medium is called:
   a) Sieving
   b) Elutriation
   c) Filtration
   d) Sedimentation
9. Which of the following factors does NOT affect the efficiency of an air classification process?
   a) Air velocity
   b) Particle density
   c) Particle shape
   d) Particle color
10. The term "cut size" in air classification refers to:
    a) The smallest particle size that can be separated
    b) The largest particle size that can be separated
    c) The particle size at which separation efficiency

is 50%

d) The average particle size of the feed material

11. Which of the following size separation techniques is most suitable for separating particles with different densities?
    a) Sieving
    b) Elutriation
    c) Filtration
    d) Magnetic separation
12. The process of separating particles based on their settling velocities in a liquid medium is called:
    a) Sieving
    b) Elutriation
    c) Sedimentation
    d) Filtration
13. Which of the following is a disadvantage of using cyclone separators?
    a) High energy consumption
    b) Inability to handle fine particles
    c) Complex equipment design
    d) Low separation efficiency for coarse particles
14. The term "screening" is most closely associated with which size separation technique?
    a) Sieving
    b) Elutriation
    c) Sedimentation
    d) Filtration
15. Which of the following factors does NOT affect the efficiency of a sedimentation process?
    a) Particle size
    b) Particle density
    c) Liquid viscosity
    d) Container material
16. The principle of differential settling is used in which of the following size separation techniques?

a) Sieving
b) Elutriation
c) Cyclone separation
d) Magnetic separation

17. Which of the following size separation techniques is most suitable for separating particles with different magnetic properties?
a) Sieving
b) Elutriation
c) Sedimentation
d) Magnetic separation

18. The process of separating particles based on their ability to be lifted by an upward flowing stream of air or liquid is called:
a) Sieving
b) Elutriation
c) Filtration
d) Cyclone separation

19. Which of the following is an advantage of wet sieving over dry sieving?
a) Lower energy consumption
b) Ability to handle heat-sensitive materials
c) More precise size separation
d) Simpler equipment design

20. The term "classification" in size separation usually refers to:
a) Separation based on particle size only
b) Separation based on particle density only
c) Separation based on both size and density
d) Separation based on particle shape only

List of Important Questions

1. What is size separation, and why is it important in pharmaceutical manufacturing?
2. Describe the different methods of size separation used in the pharmaceutical industry.
3. How does sieving work, and what are its limitations?
4. What is the principle behind air classification, and when is it preferred over sieving?
5. Explain the working principle of a cyclone separator.
6. How does elutriation contribute to size separation in pharmaceuticals?
7. What are the advantages and disadvantages of wet sieving compared to dry sieving?
8. Describe the process of sedimentation and its applications in size separation.
9. How does centrifugal sedimentation differ from gravity sedimentation?
10. What is the role of Stokes' law in size separation processes?
11. Explain the concept of cut size in classification processes.
12. How does particle shape affect the efficiency of size separation methods?
13. What are the key considerations in selecting a size separation method for a specific application?
14. Describe the principle and applications of membrane filtration in size separation.
15. How is the efficiency of a size separation process evaluated and optimized?

Bibliography

1. Allen T. Particle size measurement. 5th ed. London: Chapman & Hall; 1997.
2. Rhodes MJ. Introduction to particle technology. 2nd ed. Chichester: John Wiley & Sons; 2008.
3. Svarovsky L. Solid-liquid separation. 4th ed. Oxford: Butterworth-Heinemann; 2000.
4. Holdich RG. Fundamentals of particle technology. Shepshed: Midland Information Technology and Publishing; 2002.
5. Merkus HG. Particle size measurements: fundamentals, practice, quality. Dordrecht: Springer; 2009.
6. Aulton ME, Taylor KMG, editors. Aulton's pharmaceutics: the design and manufacture of medicines. 5th ed. Edinburgh: Elsevier; 2018.
7. Shekunov BY, Chattopadhyay P, Tong HHY, Chow AHL. Particle size analysis in pharmaceutics: principles, methods and applications. Pharm Res. 2007;24(2):203-27.
8. Staniforth JN, Aulton ME. Particle size analysis. In: Aulton ME, editor. Aulton's pharmaceutics: the design and manufacture of medicines. 3rd ed. Edinburgh: Churchill Livingstone; 2007. p. 121-37.
9. Barber TA. Pharmaceutical particulate matter: analysis and control. Buffalo Grove: Interpharm Press; 1993.
10. Seville JPK, Tüzün U, Clift R. Processing of particulate solids. London: Blackie Academic & Professional; 1997.

CHAPTER 7

MIXING

Author

Dr. Sangeetha Shanmugasundaram,
Professor, Department of Pharmaceutics, SRM College of Pharmacy, SRMIST, Kattankulathur, Tamil Nadu, India

Abstract

Mixing is a fundamental unit operation in pharmaceutical manufacturing, essential for achieving homogeneity in various formulations. This process involves the combination of two or more components to produce a uniform mixture, crucial for ensuring consistent drug content and performance. Different types of mixing are employed based on the physical state of materials, including solid-solid, solid-liquid, and liquid-liquid mixing. The selection of appropriate mixing equipment, such as ribbon blenders, planetary mixers, or high-shear mixers, depends on the nature of the materials and desired outcome. Factors affecting mixing efficiency include particle size distribution, density differences, and rheological properties of the components. The concept of mixing mechanisms, including convection, diffusion, and shear, is explored to understand the principles underlying effective mixing. Challenges in pharmaceutical mixing, such as segregation and over-mixing, are addressed, along with strategies to overcome them. Quality control measures, including blend uniformity testing and in-process controls, are discussed to ensure the consistency of the final product

Keywords: *Homogenization, Blending, Uniformity, Segregation, Mixing equipment, Process optimization*

Learning Objectives

After completion of the chapter, the student should be able to:

- Define mixing and its importance in pharmaceutical formulations.
- Explain the principles and mechanisms of mixing processes.
- Describe different types of mixing equipment used in pharmaceutical manufacturing.
- Discuss the factors affecting mixing efficiency and homogeneity.
- Explain the concept of mixing time and its optimization.
- Analyze the challenges in mixing different types of pharmaceutical materials.
- Evaluate methods for assessing the quality and uniformity of mixing.

Mixing is a critical pharmaceutical unit operation where two or more components in an unmixed or partially mixed state are combined until each unit (whether particle, molecule, or other entity) is optimally positioned adjacent to units of the other components. The theoretical pinnacle of this process is achieving a 'perfect mix,' though this ideal state is often more theoretical than practical.

Objectives of Mixing Operations

Physical Mixture Formation

The pharmaceutical industry extensively employs mixing in various dosage form preparations. This includes combining different powders or granules for tablets and capsules, blending liquids for oral solutions, and creating uniform distributions in multiple dosage forms. The primary goal is achieving homogeneous distribution of all components.

Physical Transformation

Mixing facilitates physical changes, particularly in dissolution processes. While natural diffusion can accomplish solute dissolution, mechanical agitation significantly accelerates the process. This acceleration is crucial in pharmaceutical manufacturing where time efficiency directly impacts production costs and throughput.

Dispersion Creation

In pharmaceutical dispersions like emulsions and creams, mixing serves to create stable systems where one phase is uniformly distributed throughout another. Similarly, in suspensions and pastes, solid particles must be evenly dispersed throughout a liquid medium to ensure content uniformity and product stability.

Reaction Facilitation

In pharmaceutical processes involving chemical reactions, mixing plays a dual role - it promotes uniform reaction conditions while simultaneously controlling reaction parameters to ensure consistent product quality.

Classification of Mixtures

Positive Mixtures

These systems exemplify spontaneous and irreversible mixing, typically observed with gases or miscible liquids. The process occurs naturally through diffusion without external energy input, given sufficient time. Common examples include aqueous solutions of pharmaceutical excipients, where water-soluble components distribute themselves uniformly throughout the solution.

Negative Mixtures

These systems present greater challenges as they inherently tend toward phase separation. They require continuous energy input to maintain the desired dispersed state. Many pharmaceutical suspensions fall into this category, necessitating careful formulation and mixing strategies to maintain stability.

Neutral Mixtures

These systems exhibit stability once mixed, showing neither spontaneous mixing nor separation tendencies. Many pharmaceutical semisolids and powder blends represent neutral mixtures, requiring initial energy input for mixing but maintaining their mixed state thereafter.

Solid-Solid Mixing Mechanisms

Convective Mixing

This mechanism involves the systematic movement of material masses within the mixing volume. The process occurs through mechanical means such as blade rotation, screw movement, or bed inversion, creating large-scale material redistribution.

Shear Mixing

This mechanism operates through the formation and movement of slip planes within the particle mass. The process can involve single planes or multiple parallel planes creating laminar flow patterns, effectively reducing segregation between different components.

Diffusive Mixing

This mechanism operates at the particle level, where individual particles undergo random motion and position exchange. While slower than other mechanisms, diffusive mixing is crucial for achieving microscale homogeneity, particularly at interfaces between different materials.

Equipment Considerations

Modern pharmaceutical mixing equipment must balance multiple requirements: achieving thorough mixing while minimizing product damage, maintaining cleanliness standards, preventing dust generation, and operating efficiently. Additional considerations include static charge dissipation and ease of maintenance. Tumbling mixers, specifically designed for free-flowing powders and granules, represent one common equipment category, utilizing gravitational forces and geometric design to achieve effective mixing through controlled material flow patterns

Rotating -Shell Mixers

Drum-Type Blenders

These fundamental mixing devices operate with a horizontal rotation axis through the drum's center. While widely used in pharmaceutical manufacturing, their primary limitation lies in poor axial material flow. To overcome this inherent weakness, manufacturers implement two key modifications: strategic baffle placement and axis inclination. These modifications enhance cross-flow patterns and ultimately improve mixing efficiency by creating more complex material movement patterns.

Cubical and Polyhedron Blenders

These mixers feature distinctive geometric designs with rotation axes set at various angles. While innovative in concept, polyhedron blenders face a significant operational challenge: their flat surfaces promote sliding rather than rolling motion of materials. This sliding action is less effective for achieving thorough mixing, as it fails to create the complex particle interactions necessary for uniform blending.

Double Cone Blender

The double cone design represents a significant advancement in mixing technology. Its primary advantage lies in generating superior cross-flow patterns while promoting rolling motion rather than sliding. The absence of internal baffles simplifies cleaning and maintenance procedures, making it particularly suitable for pharmaceutical applications where cross-contamination must be prevented. The geometric design naturally creates complex flow patterns that enhance mixing efficiency.

Twin Shell Blender

This sophisticated design combines two key mixing principles: the efficiency of inclined drum mixing with the advantages of split-flow patterns. The distinctive V-shaped configuration, formed by joining two cylinder halves at approximately 45 degrees, creates a unique mixing action. During operation, material alternately concentrates at the V's bottom and splits into two portions upon inversion, creating multiple opportunities for particle interaction and redistribution.

Operating Mechanism

The twin shell blender's effectiveness stems from its enhanced bulk transport and shear characteristics. The design often incorporates a counter-rotating bar with blades, intensifying powder bed agitation. This feature can be modified to accommodate liquid addition through a hollow tube, making it versatile for various pharmaceutical mixing applications.

Speed Optimization

The effectiveness of tumbling mixers critically depends on rotation speed optimization:

Low Speed Operation

Insufficient rotation speeds fail to generate adequate tumbling or cascading motion, resulting in inadequate shear rates and poor mixing performance.

High Speed Operation

Excessive speeds create problematic centrifugal forces that hold material against the mixer walls, significantly reducing mixing efficiency.

Optimal Speed Range

The ideal rotation speed typically falls between 30 to 100 rpm, though specific requirements vary based on equipment size, shape, and material characteristics.

Agitator Mixers

These systems represent an alternative approach to powder mixing, utilizing stationary containers with mobile mixing elements. While similar in concept to liquid paddle mixers, their efficiency in powder applications can be limited. However, planetary motion mixers and specialized designs offer improved performance.

Key Advantages:

- Less dependence on gravitational forces compared to tumbling mixers
- Effective handling of challenging materials like wet solids and sticky pastes
- High shear forces capable of breaking up

agglomerates and lumps.

Liquid-Solid Mixing Systems

The process of incorporating liquids into solid mixtures demands specialized equipment and techniques. When liquid must be added to powders, as in wet granulation, the mixer design must prevent the formation of agglomerates while ensuring uniform liquid distribution. The addition method plays a crucial role in achieving optimal results.

Liquid Distribution Methods

Spray addition represents the most effective approach for liquid incorporation. The liquid is typically introduced through atomizing nozzles, creating fine droplets that disperse uniformly throughout the powder mass. This method minimizes localized overwetting and helps maintain consistent granule formation. The spray pattern and droplet size must be carefully controlled to achieve optimal results.

Stream addition, while simpler, often proves less effective as it can lead to uneven wetting and lumping. This method may be suitable for very small quantities of liquid or when working with highly absorbent materials, but generally requires more mixing time and energy to achieve uniform distribution.

Mixing Equipment Selection

The choice of mixing equipment for liquid-solid systems depends largely on the properties of both phases and the desired end product characteristics. Planetary mixers excel in handling materials that become cohesive upon wetting, while high-shear mixers prove particularly effective when dealing with materials that tend to form lumps or require size reduction during the mixing process.

High Shear Mixers
These systems incorporate specially designed impellers that create intense mixing zones. The high-speed chopper blades break down agglomerates while promoting uniform liquid distribution. The bowl design typically features a rounded bottom to eliminate dead spots and ensure complete mixing. Temperature control becomes crucial in these systems due to the significant heat generation from mechanical energy input.

Planetary Mixers

Planetary mixers employ multiple mixing elements that move in both rotational and orbital patterns. This complex motion pattern proves especially effective for materials that become paste-like during mixing. The design allows for thorough scraping of bowl walls and bottom, preventing material accumulation and ensuring uniform mixing throughout the batch.

Process Control Considerations

Successful liquid-solid mixing requires careful monitoring and control of several process parameters. The rate of liquid addition must be coordinated with mixing speed and duration to prevent over-wetted regions while maintaining adequate dispersion. Temperature control becomes particularly important when working with temperature-sensitive materials or when mixing generates significant heat.

The endpoint determination in liquid-solid mixing often relies on power consumption measurements, as changes in mix consistency directly affect power requirements. Visual inspection through sight glasses or automated monitoring systems can provide additional confirmation of proper mixing progress.

Equipment Cleaning and Maintenance

The cleaning requirements for liquid-solid mixing equipment tend to be more demanding than those for dry mixing systems. Material buildup on surfaces requires thorough cleaning protocols to prevent cross-contamination between batches. Equipment design must facilitate access to all product contact surfaces while minimizing areas where material can accumulate.

Scale-up Considerations

When scaling up liquid-solid mixing operations, maintaining geometric similarity alone proves insufficient. The relationship between mixing intensity, liquid distribution, and mass transfer becomes more complex at larger scales. Successful scale-up often requires adjustments to process parameters such as liquid addition rate, mixing speed, and chopper timing to achieve comparable results to laboratory or pilot scale operations

LIQUID-LIQUID MIXING

Mixing Mechanisms

The process of liquid-liquid mixing occurs through four distinct mechanisms:

Bulk Transport Mechanism

This represents the movement of substantial liquid portions between different locations within the mixing vessel. The process involves displacement of large volumes of material, creating initial distribution patterns.

Turbulent Mixing Action

This mechanism involves random velocity fluctuations within the fluid system. The chaotic movement creates small eddies that facilitate material interchange and promote uniform distribution. These fluctuations enhance mixing efficiency by creating multiple contact opportunities between different liquid phases.

Laminar Mixing Process

In this mechanism, mixing occurs through applied shear forces that stretch the interface between dissimilar liquids. The process relies on ordered flow patterns, particularly important when dealing with viscous materials where turbulent flow is difficult to achieve.

Molecular Diffusion

The finest level of mixing occurs through molecular movement driven by thermodynamic forces. This mechanism becomes particularly significant in the final stages of mixing when achieving uniform composition at microscopic levels.

Equipment Configuration

Liquid mixing systems typically comprise two essential components:

The Mixing Element

A rotational device provides necessary shear forces and flow patterns. The design and configuration of this element significantly influence mixing effectiveness and efficiency.

The Mixing Tank

Either jacketed or non-jacketed, this vessel contains the mixing process and may include features like baffles or special geometry to enhance mixing performance.

Velocity Components

The mixing process generates three distinct velocity components:

Radial Movement

Acts perpendicular to the impeller shaft, creating horizontal material flow patterns. This component influences material distribution across the vessel diameter.

Longitudinal Flow

Operates parallel to the impeller shaft, generating vertical movement patterns. This component ensures mixing between different vertical layers within the vessel.

Tangential Motion

Creates circular movement around the impeller shaft. While necessary for mixing, excessive tangential flow can lead to undesirable vortex formation.

Flow Pattern Influences

Several factors determine the effectiveness of liquid mixing:

Equipment Configuration

The form and positioning of impellers, whether mounted centrally or offset, vertical or inclined, significantly impacts flow patterns.

Vessel Design

Container shape and internal features affect flow distribution and mixing efficiency.

Baffle Implementation

Strategic placement of baffles can prevent undesirable vortex formation and enhance mixing patterns.

Liquid Properties

The apparent viscosity of the liquids being mixed directly influences optimal operating parameters. Higher viscosity materials generally require larger impellers operating at lower speeds, while low viscosity liquids allow smaller impellers at higher speeds.

SOLID-LIQUID MIXING

Specialized Mixing Equipment for Complex Pharmaceutical Processing

Planetary Motion Mixers

The planetary mixer employs a sophisticated motion pattern mimicking planetary movement. The mixing blade simultaneously rotates on its axis while orbiting within the mixing vessel. This dual rotation creates comprehensive mixing patterns essential for challenging materials. The minimal clearance between blade and container wall prevents material accumulation and ensures thorough mixing of the entire batch.

Key applications include:

The preparation of semisolid ointments
Wet massing operations during tablet manufacturing
Processing of high-viscosity materials

Sigma Blade Mixers

Named for their distinctive sigma-shaped blades, these mixers feature dual mixing elements operating in a specialized double trough configuration. The differential speed operation, with one blade typically rotating at twice the speed of the other, creates complex material movement patterns.

Advanced features include:

Vacuum capability for air-sensitive materials

Temperature control through jacketed vessels and hollow blades

Enhanced mixing through differential blade speeds

Robust construction for heavy-duty applications

Triple Roller Mill Technology

This specialized equipment excels in particle size reduction and material incorporation for semisolid preparations. The system employs three precisely aligned rollers operating at different speeds with progressively decreasing gaps between them.

Operating sequence:

Material feeds through initial rollers for preliminary size reduction

Secondary rolling provides further refinement

Final rolling achieves ultimate particle size and mixture smoothness

Continuous scraping ensures efficient material collection

Homogenization Systems

Homogenizers utilize high-pressure processing to achieve uniform dispersion and particle size reduction. The process involves forcing material through specialized valve assemblies under controlled conditions.

Operating principles:

Materials enter under high pressure (1000-5000 psi)

Rapid pressure drops create intense shear forces

Impact ring contact provides additional particle disruption

Optional two-stage processing prevents particle reagglomeration

Two-Stage Homogenization Process:

First stage: High-pressure processing (3000-5000 psi)

Second stage: Reduced pressure processing (approximately 1000 psi)

This sequential approach prevents cluster formation and enhances stability

Implementation Strategies:

Direct processing of complete formulation

Secondary processing of pre-mixed systems

Selection depends on specific product requirements and material characteristics

Process Control Considerations

Each mixing system requires careful attention to:

Processing parameters

Temperature management

Material characteristics

End-point determination

Equipment maintenance requirements.

SILVERSON EMULSIFIER

Principle

Silverson mixer emulsifiers use high-speed rotors to create turbulence and intense shearing forces. Through the turbulence created by the perforated metal sheets, the liquid passes through fine interstices. Suction from the bottom of the head causes material to circulate through the head. The dispersed liquid is rapidly broken down into smaller globules because of the circulation of the material.

Construction

The figure depicts the process of constructing a Silverson emulsifier. A motor attached to long columns provides support to the head. A shaft runs through the center of the machine, with one end connected to the motor and the other to the head. Turbine blades are attached to the head. In addition to the mesh surrounding the blades, there is a cover with openings that surrounds them

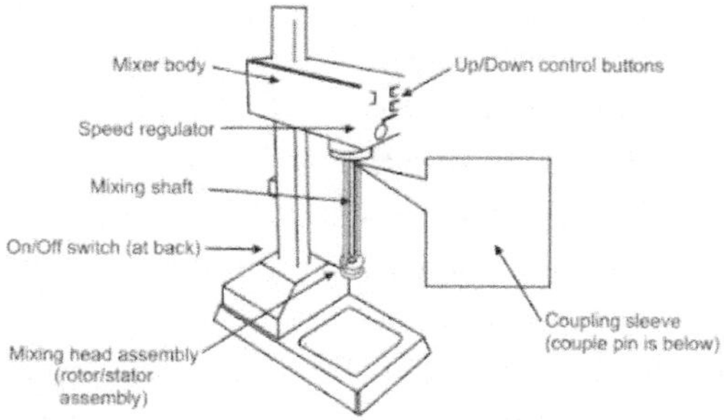

Working

Emulsifier heads are introduced into vessels containing immiscible liquids (or coarse emulsions) in such a way that they are fully submerged in the liquid. Motors rotate the head with the help of the central rotating shaft, which in turn spins turbine blades at high speeds. The result is a pressure differential. Consequently, liquids are drawn into the head of the device from the base, where they are mixed vigorously. In a centrifugal fashion, the contents of the head are pushed out of the head through the mesh and onto the cover (Figure). Through the outer cover openings, a fine emulsion emerges. As the mixture is taken in and expelled, a pattern develops that facilitates the breakdown of the larger globules into smaller ones.

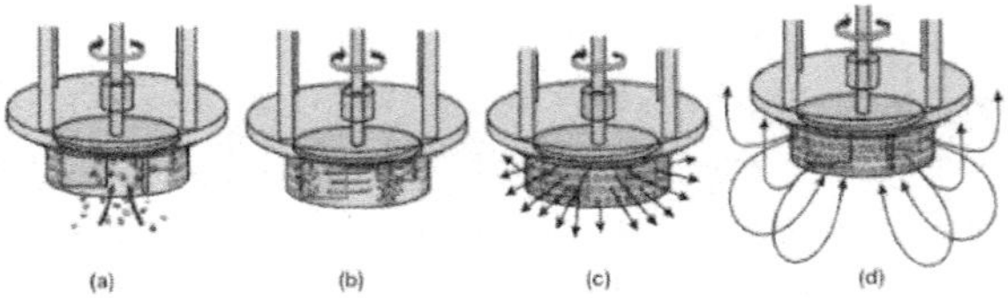

Uses

- Solids can be mixed, emulsified, homogenized, dissolved, suspended, dispersed, and disintegrated using it.
- Emulsions between 0.5 and 5 microns are prepared using this device.
- The Silverson mixer can disintegrate matter from any source, including animal, vegetable, mineral, and synthetic sources.
- Solid and semi-solid materials can be uniformly ground into solution or fine suspensions with the aid of this equipment.
- Rapid gelling is also possible with it. The solubilization and dispersing of gums, alginates, CMCs, carbopols, etc., leading to agglomerate-free solutions in minutes.

Merits

- Mixing times can be reduced by up to 90% with this efficient, fast machine.
- Shear mixers are efficient, aeration-free, fast, reliable, and versatile.
- Typically, it produces micron-sized droplets or particles, usually between 2 and 5 microns.
- It reduces operating costs by being efficient.
- Homogenizers normally pass the product more

quickly; normally in a single pass.
- Mixing applications can be performed with this versatile device thanks to its versatility.

Demerits
- Premixed feeds should have fine globules or particles that are uniform in size.
- It consumes more energy.

COLLOID MILL

Operational Principles

The colloid mill achieves particle size reduction and dispersion through intense shearing forces generated between a high-speed rotor and fixed stator assembly. The rotor operates at exceptionally high speeds ranging from 2,000 to 18,000 rpm, creating powerful shear zones in the processing area.

Critical Design Elements

Rotor-Stator Configuration

Precise clearance adjustment between components (starting at 0.001 inch)

Variable speed control systems

Temperature management features

Process monitoring capabilities

Operating Parameters

Speed Range Control

Adjustable clearance settings

Temperature monitoring

Flow rate regulation
Material feed consistency

Thermal Management

The intense mechanical energy input generates significant heat during operation. Temperature control systems typically include:

Cooling jacket integration

Heat exchanger systems
Temperature monitoring devices
Automated cooling control mechanisms

Performance Advantages

Exceptional Shear Force Generation
Superior particle size reduction capability
Uniform particle size distribution
Enhanced processing of difficult-to-wet materials
Excellent performance with viscous emulsions

Process Applications

Primary Processing
Emulsion preparation
Suspension processing
Particle size reduction
Material dispersion

Specialized Uses

Processing poorly wettable solids
High-viscosity emulsion formation
Fine particle generation
Uniform dispersion creation.

Summary

Mixing is a fundamental unit operation in pharmaceutical manufacturing, essential for achieving homogeneity in multi-component systems and ensuring uniform distribution of active ingredients and excipients. This process involves the intermingling of two or more components to produce a uniform product, critical for maintaining consistent drug quality and efficacy. Various types of mixing are employed in pharmaceutical production, including solid-solid, liquid-liquid, and solid-liquid mixing, each with unique challenges and methodologies. Solid-solid mixing, common in powder blending for tablet and capsule formulations, utilizes equipment such as tumble blenders, ribbon blenders, and high-shear mixers. Liquid-liquid mixing, crucial in the preparation of solutions and emulsions, employs stirred tanks, static mixers, and homogenizers. Solid-liquid mixing, essential for suspension and slurry preparation, often involves specialized impeller designs and baffled vessels. The efficiency of mixing is influenced by factors including particle size distribution, density differences, cohesiveness, and rheological properties of the materials. Mixing mechanisms involve convection (bulk material movement), diffusion (random motion of particles), and shear (relative movement between adjacent layers). The choice of mixing equipment and parameters depends on the physical properties of the materials, batch size, and desired end-product characteristics. Continuous mixing processes are gaining prominence in pharmaceutical manufacturing, offering advantages in terms of consistency and scalability. Evaluation of mixing effectiveness involves sampling techniques and analytical methods to assess content uniformity and blend homogeneity. Challenges in pharmaceutical mixing include preventing segregation in powder blends, maintaining stability of shear-sensitive materials, and ensuring complete dispersion of minor components. Computational fluid dynamics (CFD) and process analytical technology (PAT) are increasingly used to optimize mixing processes and ensure robust, consistent results. Proper mixing is crucial for downstream processing and ultimately impacts the quality, safety, and efficacy of the final pharmaceutical product.

Multiple Choice Questions

1. What is the primary purpose of mixing in pharmaceutical manufacturing?
   a) To increase particle size
   b) To achieve uniform distribution of components
   c) To reduce moisture content
   d) To increase bulk density
2. Which of the following is NOT a type of mixing?
   a) Solid-solid mixing
   b) Liquid-liquid mixing
   c) Gas-gas mixing
   d) Crystal-crystal mixing
3. The term "dead spots" in mixing refers to:
   a) Areas where mixing is most efficient
   b) Regions of stagnant material
   c) Points where mixing speed is highest
   d) Zones of maximum shear
4. Which type of mixer is most suitable for mixing viscous liquids?
   a) Ribbon blender
   b) Tumbling mixer
   c) Planetary mixer
   d) Fluidized bed mixer

5. The principle of convection is primarily used in which type of mixer?
   a) Ribbon blender
   b) High shear mixer
   c) V-blender
   d) Sigma blade mixer
6. Which of the following factors does NOT affect mixing efficiency?
   a) Mixer speed
   b) Batch size
   c) Mixing time
   d) Operator's experience
7. What is the main advantage of using a high shear mixer?
   a) Low energy consumption
   b) Gentle mixing action
   c) Rapid mixing of cohesive powders
   d) Large batch capacity
8. The process of mixing where particles are redistributed by the movement of large groups of particles is called:
   a) Convection
   b) Diffusion
   c) Shear
   d) Tumbling
9. Which type of mixer is most suitable for mixing heat-sensitive materials?
   a) High shear mixer
   b) Ribbon blender
   c) Tumbling mixer
   d) Planetary mixer
10. The term "segregation" in mixing refers to:
   a) Uniform distribution of particles
   b) Separation of particles based on size or density

c) Agglomeration of particles
d) Reduction in particle size

11. Which of the following is an example of a continuous mixer?
a) V-blender
b) Ribbon blender
c) Planetary mixer
d) Tumbling mixer
12. The principle of diffusion in mixing is most effective for:
a) Large particles
b) Cohesive powders
c) Fine particles
d) Wet granulations
13. Which type of mixer is most suitable for mixing small quantities of potent drugs with larger quantities of excipients?
a) Ribbon blender
b) High shear mixer
c) Geometric dilution method
d) Fluidized bed mixer
14. The term "critical speed" in tumbling mixers refers to:
a) The maximum speed at which the mixer can operate
b) The speed at which material starts to centrifuge
c) The minimum speed required for mixing
d) The speed at which the mixer consumes the least energy
15. Which of the following factors contributes to increased mixing time?
a) Decreased particle size difference
b) Increased mixer speed
c) Decreased batch size
d) Increased cohesiveness of powders.

List of Important Questions

1. What is mixing, and why is it crucial in pharmaceutical manufacturing?
2. Describe the different types of mixing processes used in pharmaceuticals.
3. What are the main mechanisms involved in solid-solid mixing?
4. How does liquid-liquid mixing differ from solid-liquid mixing in terms of process and equipment?
5. Explain the concept of mixing efficiency and how it is measured.
6. What factors affect the homogeneity of a mixture in pharmaceutical processing?
7. Describe the working principle of a ribbon blender and its applications.
8. How does a high shear mixer work, and when is it preferred in pharmaceutical formulations?
9. What are the advantages and limitations of tumbling mixers?
10. Explain the importance of scaling up mixing processes in pharmaceutical manufacturing.
11. How does the order of addition of ingredients affect the mixing process and final product quality?
12. What are the key considerations in mixing heat-sensitive or moisture-sensitive materials?
13. Describe the role of mixing in achieving content uniformity in solid dosage forms.
14. How is mixing time determined and optimized in pharmaceutical processes?
15. What are the latest innovations in mixing technology for pharmaceuticals?

Bibliography

1. Harnby N, Edwards MF, Nienow AW. Mixing in the process industries. 2nd ed. Oxford: Butterworth-Heinemann; 1997.
2. Paul EL, Atiemo-Obeng VA, Kresta SM, editors. Handbook of industrial mixing: science and practice. Hoboken: John Wiley & Sons; 2004.
3. Muzzio FJ, Alexander A, Goodridge C, Shen E, Shinbrot T, Manjunath K, et al. Solids mixing. In: Atiemo-Obeng VA, Calabrese RV, editors. Advances in industrial mixing: a companion to the handbook of industrial mixing. Hoboken: John Wiley & Sons; 2016. p. 887-985.
4. Bridgwater J. Mixing of powders and granular materials by mechanical means—a perspective. Particuology. 2012;10(4):397-427.
5. Fan LT, Chen YM, Lai FS. Recent developments in solids mixing. Powder Technol. 1990;61(3):255-87.
6. Poux M, Fayolle P, Bertrand J, Bridoux D, Bousquet J. Powder mixing: some practical rules applied to agitated systems. Powder Technol. 1991;68(3):213-34.
7. Weinekötter R, Gericke H. Mixing of solids. Dordrecht: Kluwer Academic Publishers; 2000.
8. Ortega-Rivas E. Mixing and segregation. In: Ortega-Rivas E, editor. Unit operations of particulate solids: theory and practice. Boca Raton: CRC Press; 2012. p. 155-98.
9. Jain A, Metzger MJ, Glasser BJ. Effect of particle size distribution on segregation in vibrated systems. Powder Technol. 2013;237:543-53.
10. Brone D, Muzzio FJ. Enhanced mixing in double-cone blenders. Powder Technol. 2000;110(3):179-89.

CHAPTER 8

FILTRATION

Author

Mrs. Parimala Vudikala
Assistant Professor, Department of Pharmaceutics, Joginpally BR Pharmacy College, Moinabad, Hyderabad, Telangana, India

Abstract

Filtration is a critical separation process in pharmaceutical manufacturing used to remove solid particles from liquids or gases. This operation is essential for purifying raw materials, intermediate products, and final drug formulations. Various filtration mechanisms, including surface straining, depth filtration, and cake filtration, are employed depending on the nature of the suspension and desired level of separation. The selection of appropriate filter media, such as membrane filters, depth filters, or cartridge filters, is crucial for achieving optimal filtration efficiency. Factors influencing filtration performance include particle size distribution, filter pore size, pressure differential, and filtration rate. The principles of constant pressure and constant rate filtration are explored, along with their applications in different pharmaceutical processes. Advanced filtration techniques, such as tangential flow filtration and sterile filtration, are discussed in the context of biotechnology products and aseptic processing. Quality control measures, including integrity testing of sterilizing filters and validation of filtration processes, are essential to ensure product sterility and purity. Understanding filtration principles and practices is vital for maintaining product quality and compliance with regulatory standards in pharmaceutical manufacturing

Keywords: *Separation, Filter media, Particle retention, Sterile filtration, Cake formation, Process validation*

Learning Objectives

After completion of the chapter, the student should be able to:

- Define filtration and its role in pharmaceutical processing.
- Explain the principles and mechanisms of filtration.
- Describe different types of filters and filtration equipment used in pharmaceuticals.
- Discuss the factors affecting filtration efficiency and rate.
- Explain the concept of filter aids and their applications.
- Analyze the challenges in filtering different types of pharmaceutical solutions and suspensions.
- Evaluate methods for assessing the quality and effectiveness of filtration processes.

Basic Components

The filtration process involves four key components. The slurry represents the initial solid-liquid suspension requiring separation. The filter medium serves as the porous barrier designed to retain solids while allowing liquid passage. As filtration progresses, the filter cake develops as an accumulation of retained solids on the medium surface. The filtrate emerges as the clarified liquid that has successfully passed through both the filter medium and cake layers.

Primary Filtration Mechanisms

Initial Particle Retention

The initial phase of filtration employs multiple mechanisms for particle capture. Straining occurs when particles are physically too large to pass through the medium pores. Impingement captures particles through their inertial collision with filter fibers when they deviate from fluid streamlines. Entanglement takes place as particles become trapped within the complex fiber network of the filter medium. Attractive forces, particularly electrostatic interactions, can bind particles to the filter surface through charge-based mechanisms.

Kozeny's Equation Filtration

Once the initial particle layer forms, the filtration process transitions to cake filtration, governed by Kozeny's equation. This mathematical relationship describes flow rate (dV/dt) as a function of pressure differential (P), filtration area (A), fluid viscosity (μ), and total system resistance (R). This equation becomes the primary model for understanding and predicting filtration behavior in established systems.

Critical Process Factors

Medium and Cake Properties

The filter medium's inherent resistance plays a crucial role in initial filtration stages, though its importance diminishes relative to cake resistance in prolonged operations. Cake properties, including thickness, particle size distribution, shape characteristics, and material compressibility, significantly influence filtration efficiency. Filter aids may be necessary for compressible materials to maintain adequate flow rates.

Operating Parameters

Filtration area directly impacts processing capacity,

with larger areas enabling higher throughput. Pressure differential drives the filtration process, while fluid viscosity affects flow resistance. The progressive development of cake thickness requires careful monitoring and management to maintain efficient operation.

Pressure Generation Methods

Gravity Systems

Gravity-based filtration offers simplicity and reliability, utilizing the hydrostatic pressure of the slurry column. While straightforward to operate and maintain, these systems are limited by achievable pressure differentials.

Vacuum Systems

Vacuum filtration provides controlled pressure differentials through reduced pressure below the filter medium. Though effective, these systems are limited to one atmosphere of pressure differential and may experience complications with volatile liquids.

Positive Pressure

Positive pressure systems enable higher pressure differentials through direct pressurization of the slurry. This approach offers superior control and capability but requires more complex equipment and maintenance.

Centrifugal Systems

Centrifugal filtration generates separation forces through rotation, enabling continuous operation and high efficiency. While offering excellent performance, these systems involve higher capital costs and operational complexity.

Filter Media Classifications

Surface Filtration

Surface filtration media include screen type, edge type, and stacked disc configurations. These media primarily function through surface capture of particles larger than their openings, offering precise particle size cutoff but potentially limited capacity.

Depth Filtration

Depth filtration employs fibrous, porous, and cake-type media. These materials capture particles throughout their structure rather than just on the surface, providing higher capacity and efficiency for certain applications but potentially more complex flow patterns and cleaning requirements.

Process Optimization

Successful filtration requires careful attention to temperature control for managing fluid viscosity, proper pre-filtration concentration adjustment, and implementation of appropriate cake removal strategies. System design must balance filtration area, pressure differential, and medium selection to achieve optimal performance while maintaining economic operation

SURFACE FILTRATION MEDIA

Screen Type Media

Screen type filtration media encompasses a diverse range of materials crafted into specialized cloths. These materials include natural fibers like wool, cotton, and silk, as well as synthetic options such as rayon and nylon, and inorganic materials like glass and metals. Muslin cloth, made from cotton with duck weave, provides excellent porosity and surface hardness, though it shows vulnerability to chemical attack. Nitrated cotton offers enhanced surface hardness, while glass cloth delivers superior thermal and corrosion resistance alongside high tensile strength, despite limited flexibility. Synthetic materials, particularly nylon, demonstrate excellent chemical resistance and thermal stability, with the added benefit of resistance to microbial growth. Metallic screens, constructed from various metals including steel, copper, bronze, and nickel, excel in handling corrosive substances and high-temperature applications.

Edge Type Media

Edge type filtration employs a specialized cartridge design where fluid flows from the exterior to the interior. The construction consists of compressed discs or washers, which may be made from paper, plastic, or metal. These components feature spacing projections that create controlled channels between discs. This design enables efficient solid particle retention on the outer surface, where regular cleaning can be performed. The system maintains consistent performance during pressure fluctuations and resists clogging, making it particularly reliable for continuous operations.

Stacked Disc Filters

This configuration features individual discs arranged around a central perforated tube, separated by precise spacing washers. The design creates a uniform filtration surface while maintaining structural integrity throughout the filtration process.

DEPTH FILTRATION MEDIA

Fibrous Medium

Depth filtration through fibrous media utilizes randomly oriented fibers creating complex pathways for particle capture. These media incorporate materials such as cotton, cellulose, rayon, polypropylene, and micro-glass fibers. Resin binding ensures structural integrity during operation. Notably, electret filter media, comprising permanently charged dielectric polymers, offers enhanced particle collection efficiency with minimal pressure drop, making them ideal for clean air applications in medical and pharmaceutical environments. Borosilicate microfibers, fused through heat and pressure, provide exceptional chemical resistance.

Porous Medium

Porous filtration media consist of sintered materials including glass, metals, plastics, or ceramics. These materials create intricate capillary networks, with adjustable pore sizes to match specific filtration requirements.

FILTER AIDS

Function and Mechanism

Filter aids serve to enhance filtration efficiency when processing highly compressible materials. These additives, typically used in concentrations up to 5%, reduce cake resistance by creating more rigid and porous structures. Their irregular shape, controlled surface area, and narrow particle size distribution provide essential support for compressible particles.

Common Materials

Various materials serve as filter aids, including purified talc, diatomaceous earth, charcoal, kaolin, asbestos, cellulose, and pearlite. Each material offers specific advantages depending on the application requirements.

Concentration Effects

The relationship between filter aid concentration and filtration rate follows a distinctive pattern. Initial increases in concentration improve filtration rates through enhanced porosity. However, beyond an optimal concentration, increased cake thickness begins to dominate, resulting in reduced filtration rates. This balance between porosity and thickness determines the optimal filter aid concentration.

Application Methods

Filter aids can be applied through three primary methods. The body mix method involves direct incorporation into the slurry. The pre-coat method establishes a preliminary filter aid layer before main filtration begins. The special pre-coat method, specifically designed for rotary drum filters, combines both approaches while maintaining precise control over cake removal

DEPTH FILTRATION MEDIA

Depth filtration media are engineered with a gradient density structure, becoming progressively denser from the outer to inner layers. This design optimizes particle capture throughout the medium's depth.

Fibrous Medium

Fibrous media consist of intricately arranged fine fibers forming a complex mat structure. These fibers, which may include cotton, cellulose, rayon, polypropylene, and micro-glass fibers, create tortuous pathways that effectively trap particles. The structural integrity is maintained through resin bonding of the fiber layers. A notable advancement in this category is the electret filter medium, which incorporates permanently charged dielectric polymers. This technology creates an open structure that achieves high collection efficiency while maintaining low pressure drop, making it particularly valuable in healthcare and pharmaceutical environments for air purification. Borosilicate microfibers, produced through heat and pressure fusion, offer additional benefits through their superior chemical resistance.

Porous Medium

Porous filtration media utilize sintered materials including glass, metals, plastics, and ceramics. These materials create interconnected capillary networks whose pore sizes can be precisely controlled to match specific filtration requirements.

FILTER AIDS

Basic Principles

Filter aids become essential when processing slurries containing highly compressible materials, which typically form cakes with excessive flow resistance. These additives, used in concentrations up to 5%, effectively reduce cake resistance and enhance filtration rates.

Mechanism of Action

The effectiveness of filter aids stems from their unique physical characteristics. Their irregular shape, combined with low surface area and narrow particle size distribution, creates a rigid framework within the filter cake. This structure maintains porosity and provides crucial support for compressible particles.

Common Filter Aid Materials

The range of filter aids includes purified talc, diatomaceous earth (keiselghur), charcoal, kaolin, asbestos, cellulose, and pearlite (volcanic glass). Each material offers specific advantages for different applications.

Concentration Effects on Filtration

The relationship between filter aid concentration and filtration performance follows a predictable pattern. Initially, increasing concentration improves filtration rates as cake porosity increases. However, an optimal point exists where maximum filtration efficiency is achieved. Beyond this point, the increased cake thickness begins to dominate, resulting in decreased filtration rates.

Application Methods

Body Mix Method

This technique involves directly incorporating filter aid into the slurry at concentrations between 0.01% and 4% w/v before filtration.

Pre-coat Method

When dealing with high pressure drops, this method involves creating an initial filter aid layer before introducing the main slurry.

Special Pre-coat Method

This specialized technique, designed for rotary drum filters, involves forming a filter aid pre-coat without the scraper knife, followed by main slurry filtration with the scraper knife in place, which removes both the cake and a thin layer of pre-coat.

INDUSTRIAL FILTERS

1. Leaf filters
2. Filter press
3. Rotary filters e.g. Rotary drum filter
4. Edge filters e.g. Meta filter

Leaf Filters

A leaf filter consists of a frame housing a drainage screen or grooved plate covered with filter cloth. The filtrate outlet connects directly to the frame, which can be circular, square, or rectangular in shape. During operation, the assembly is submerged in slurry under vacuum, causing solids to accumulate on the cloth while filtrate passes through the outlet. Cake washing is accomplished by immersing the filter in water and applying reverse airflow.

Sweetland Filter

The Sweetland filter represents an advanced leaf filter design, incorporating multiple filter leaves within a cylindrical vessel. Its split design features a fixed upper section and a movable lower portion. This configuration allows pressure differences up to 8 bars and offers excellent washing efficiency. However, its operation is limited to slurries with concentrations below 5% w/v.

Chamber Press

The chamber press employs corrugated filter plates positioned between two fixed cast iron heads. These plates, supported by lugs on extending rods, feature central holes for feed introduction. Filter cloth sheets with central holes are secured using grommets. The assembly is compressed either by screw mechanism or hydraulic pressure, with the cloths acting as gaskets between plates.

Plate-Frame Filter Press

This design alternates plates and frames, with plates featuring raised edges and corrugated surfaces, while frames are hollow structures ranging from 2 to 15 cm in thickness. Available in both non-washing and washing types, these filters can handle various materials through different collection systems. The non-washing type utilizes a single corner hole design, while the washing type incorporates multiple holes for thorough cake cleaning.

Advantages and Applications

Plate-frame presses offer remarkable versatility in construction materials, including cast iron, bronze, stainless steel, and plastics. They provide substantial filtering area in minimal floor space and can withstand pressures up to 20 bars. Common applications include bismuth salt filtration and protein precipitation separation in pharmaceutical processes.

Rotary Filters

Rotary filters feature a hollow metal cylinder with mesh support for filter cloth, operating in distinct zones including pick-up, drainage, washing, drying, and cake removal. Available in sizes up to 2m diameter and 3.5m length, these filters rotate at 0.1-3 rpm. Cake discharge occurs through scrapper, string, or belt mechanisms.

Operational Characteristics

These filters excel in continuous operation with high capacity, handling slurries containing 15-30% solids. Speed adjustment allows precise cake thickness control, ranging from 5mm for impenetrable cakes to 100mm for porous materials. Primary applications include calcium carbonate separation and antibiotic fermentation processing.

Limitations and Considerations

While rotary filters offer automation advantages, their complex design and high cost pose significant considerations. They face challenges with vacuum-induced cake cracking and are unsuitable for near-boiling liquids. Additionally, gelatinous precipitates may present separation difficulties from the filter cloth

EDGE FILTER

Edge filters employ a unique filtration mechanism utilizing a stack of filter media where filtration occurs along the edges. The design incorporates multiple metal rings arranged on a fluted rod, with the rod's surface grooves facilitating filtrate discharge. These rings, typically constructed from stainless steel, feature precise dimensions - 15mm internal diameter, 22mm external diameter, and 0.8mm thickness. The plate design incorporates semicircular projections that, when assembled, create tapered channels ranging from 250 to 25 micrometers.

Metafilter Construction and Operation

The metafilter assembly consists of multiple filter packs mounted within a vessel. Filtration occurs through either pressure pumping or vacuum application. The system allows cake removal through water backflushing or mechanical scraping. This design offers exceptional durability, enabling high-pressure operation without compromising filter medium integrity. The elimination of traditional filter media reduces operational costs significantly.

Membrane Filter Systems

Membrane filters represent advanced filtration technology, featuring microporous surfaces with pore sizes ranging from 0.005 to 12 micrometers. These filters utilize various materials including cellulose acetate, cellulose nitrates, PTFE, PVC, and nylon. Available in both disc and cartridge configurations, these systems accommodate membrane diameters from 13 to 293 millimeters.

Operational Protocols

The membrane filtration process begins with water-soaking the membrane before installation in the filter holder. Filtration proceeds either through vacuum application from the filtrate side or positive pressure from the slurry side. Filter longevity remains limited due to clogging issues, particularly when processing thick solutions or fibrous materials like blood, gelatin, or plant extracts.

Integrity Testing Procedures

Membrane filter integrity assessment involves two primary methods. The bubble-point test determines pore characteristics by measuring the pressure required to force liquid from capillaries. The bacterial challenge test evaluates filter effectiveness by passing specific bacterial cultures through the membrane and monitoring subsequent growth.

Filter Selection Criteria

Selection considerations include filtration purpose, operating conditions, and process requirements. Purpose-specific applications range from solid collection and filtrate recovery to air purification and sterilization. Operating parameters encompass pore size requirements, chemical compatibility, temperature limitations, and particle concentration levels.

SINTERED GLASS FILTER

These filters operate on pressure differential principles, utilizing a glass funnel with a sintered disc construction. The filtering medium consists of uniformly sized glass granules molded together, offering various porosity levels. Operation typically requires vacuum assistance for liquid passage through the filter plate.

Advantages and Limitations

Each filtration system presents distinct benefits and challenges. Edge filters and metafilters excel in high-pressure applications and offer low operating costs. Membrane filters provide precise filtration but face clogging issues. Sintered glass filters offer excellent chemical resistance but remain fragile and costly.

Application

The selection of appropriate filtration technology depends heavily on specific application requirements. Factors including particle size, solution characteristics, required throughput, and operational conditions determine optimal filter selection. Understanding these parameters ensures effective filtration system implementation.

Future Developments

Ongoing technological advancements continue to enhance filtration capabilities. Innovations in materials science and design engineering promise improved efficiency, durability, and operational flexibility across all filtration technologies. These developments address current limitations while expanding application possibilities.

Summary

Filtration is a critical separation process in pharmaceutical manufacturing, used to remove solid particles from liquids or gases, ensuring product purity and sterility. This operation relies on the principle of size exclusion, where a porous medium retains particles larger than its pore size while allowing the fluid to pass through. Various filtration methods are employed, each suited to specific applications and particle size ranges. Depth filtration utilizes thick, porous media to trap particles throughout its structure, commonly used for clarification of liquids with high particle loads. Surface filtration, including membrane filtration, captures particles on the filter surface and is preferred for sterile filtration of parenteral products. Cake filtration involves the build-up of retained solids on the filter surface, forming an additional filtration layer. Equipment used in pharmaceutical filtration includes plate and frame filters, cartridge filters, and tangential flow filtration systems. The choice of filter media is crucial, with options ranging from cellulose-based materials to synthetic polymers and inorganic membranes, each offering different chemical compatibility and retention characteristics. Filtration efficiency is influenced by factors such as particle size distribution, fluid viscosity, temperature, and pressure differential across the filter. Sterilizing-grade filters, typically with a pore size of 0.2 μm or smaller, are essential for removing microorganisms from heat-sensitive solutions. Integrity testing of sterilizing filters, using methods like bubble point test and diffusive flow test, is critical to ensure filter performance. Challenges in pharmaceutical filtration include membrane fouling, which can reduce filtration efficiency and throughput, and the potential for extractables and leachables from filter materials. Advanced filtration technologies, such as nanofiltration and ultrafiltration, are increasingly used for specific applications like virus removal and protein purification. Process analytical technology (PAT) is employed to monitor filtration processes in real-time, optimizing performance and ensuring consistent product quality. Proper selection and validation of filtration processes are essential to meet regulatory requirements and maintain product safety and efficacy.

Multiple Choice Questions

1. What is the primary purpose of filtration in pharmaceutical manufacturing?
   a) To mix components
   b) To separate solids from liquids
   c) To reduce particle size
   d) To increase solubility
2. Which of the following is NOT a type of filtration?
   a) Surface filtration
   b) Depth filtration

c) Cake filtration
d) Molecular filtration

3. The term "filter medium" refers to:
a) The liquid being filtered
b) The porous material that retains solids
c) The equipment used for filtration
d) The solid particles being removed
4. Which type of filter is most suitable for sterile filtration of liquids?
a) Plate and frame filter
b) Membrane filter
c) Rotary drum filter
d) Nutsche filter
5. The principle of centrifugal force is used in which type of filter?
a) Basket centrifuge
b) Cartridge filter
c) Leaf filter
d) Belt filter
6. Which of the following factors does NOT affect filtration rate?
a) Viscosity of the liquid
b) Pressure difference across the filter
c) Filter medium porosity
d) Color of the filtrate
7. What is the main advantage of using a continuous rotary vacuum filter?
a) Low energy consumption
b) High filtration efficiency for viscous liquids
c) Ability to handle large volumes continuously
d) Suitability for sterile filtration
8. The process of filtration where particles are trapped within the depth of the filter medium is called:
a) Surface filtration

b) Depth filtration
c) Cake filtration
d) Cross-flow filtration

9. Which type of filter is most suitable for filtration of heat-sensitive materials?
a) Plate and frame filter
b) Rotary drum filter
c) Membrane filter
d) Nutsche filter

10. The term "filter aid" refers to:
a) A chemical that enhances filtration
b) A material added to improve filtration efficiency
c) The equipment used for filtration
d) The pressure applied during filtration

11. Which of the following is an example of a depth filter?
a) Membrane filter
b) Sintered glass filter
c) Wire mesh filter
d) Paper filter

12. The principle of tangential flow is used in which type of filtration?
a) Dead-end filtration
b) Cross-flow filtration
c) Cake filtration
d) Depth filtration

13. Which type of filter is most suitable for clarifying large volumes of liquid with low solid content?
a) Plate and frame filter
b) Cartridge filter
c) Nutsche filter
d) Belt filter

14. The term "filter cake" refers to:
a) The liquid that passes through the filter

b) The layer of solids that accumulates on the filter surface
c) The filter medium itself
d) The equipment used for filtration

15. Which of the following factors contributes to increased filtration efficiency?
a) Increased particle size of solids
b) Decreased pressure difference
c) Increased viscosity of liquid
d) Decreased filter medium porosity

List of Important Questions

1. What is filtration, and why is it important in pharmaceutical manufacturing?
2. Describe the different types of filtration processes used in the pharmaceutical industry.
3. What are the main components of a filtration system?
4. Explain the concept of filter media and how it affects filtration efficiency.
5. How does cake filtration differ from depth filtration?
6. What is the role of Darcy's law in understanding filtration processes?
7. Describe the working principle of a plate and frame filter press.
8. How does a rotary drum filter operate, and what are its applications in pharmaceuticals?
9. What are the advantages and limitations of membrane filtration?
10. Explain the concept of filter aid and its role in improving filtration efficiency.
11. How does the particle size distribution of a suspension affect the filtration process?

12. Describe the challenges in filtration of viscous liquids and how they are addressed.
13. What are the key considerations in selecting a filtration method for sterile products?
14. How is the efficiency of a filtration process evaluated and optimized?
15. What are the latest innovations in filtration technology for pharmaceuticals?

Bibliography

1. Wakeman RJ, Tarleton ES. Filtration: equipment selection, modelling and process simulation. Oxford: Elsevier; 1999.
2. Sutherland K. Filters and filtration handbook. 5th ed. Oxford: Butterworth-Heinemann; 2008.
3. Tien C. Introduction to cake filtration: analyses, experiments and applications. Amsterdam: Elsevier; 2006.
4. Rushton A, Ward AS, Holdich RG. Solid-liquid filtration and separation technology. 2nd ed. Weinheim: Wiley-VCH; 2000.
5. Cheremisinoff NP. Liquid filtration. 2nd ed. Boston: Butterworth-Heinemann; 1998.
6. Sparks T, Chase G. Filters and filtration handbook. 6th ed. Oxford: Butterworth-Heinemann; 2016.
7. Wakeman RJ. Selection of equipment for solid/liquid separation processes. Filtr Sep. 1995;32(4):337-41.
8. Tarleton ES, Wakeman RJ. Solid/liquid separation: equipment selection and process design. Oxford: Elsevier; 2007.
9. Tiller FM, Yeh CS, Tsai CD. Theory of filtration of ceramics: I. Slip casting. J Am Ceram Soc. 1987;70(6):372-9.

10. Dickenson TC. Filters and filtration handbook. 4th ed. Oxford: Elsevier Advanced Technology; 1997.

CHAPTER 9

DRYING

Author

Dr. Syed Afzal Uddin Biyabani,
Research Scholar, Rajiv Gandhi University of Health Sciences, Bangalore, India

Abstract

Drying is a crucial unit operation in pharmaceutical manufacturing, involving the removal of moisture or other solvents from solid, semi-solid, or liquid materials. This process is essential for enhancing the stability, handling properties, and shelf life of pharmaceutical products. Various drying mechanisms, including evaporation, vaporization, and sublimation, are employed depending on the nature of the material and desired end-product characteristics. Different types of dryers, such as tray dryers, fluidized bed dryers, spray dryers, and freeze dryers, are used based on the specific requirements of the formulation. Factors affecting drying efficiency include heat and mass transfer rates, material properties, and equipment design. The concept of drying kinetics, including constant rate and falling rate periods, is explored to understand the drying process dynamics. Critical process parameters, such as inlet air temperature, airflow rate, and product bed depth, are discussed in relation to their impact on product quality. Special considerations for heat-sensitive materials and the drying of hygroscopic substances are addressed. Quality control measures, including moisture content determination and uniformity testing, are essential to ensure consistent product quality

Keywords: *Moisture removal, Solvent evaporation, Drying kinetics, Stability enhancement, Lyophilization, Process optimization*

Learning Objectives

After completion of the chapter, the student should be able to:

- Define drying and its importance in pharmaceutical manufacturing.
- Explain the principles and mechanisms of various drying processes.
- Describe different types of drying equipment used in pharmaceuticals.
- Discuss the factors affecting drying efficiency and product quality.
- Explain the concept of moisture content and its measurement techniques.
- Analyze the impact of drying on drug stability and properties.
- Evaluate methods for optimizing drying processes in pharmaceutical production.

Drying represents a thermal process for liquid removal from solids, distinct from evaporation which handles larger liquid volumes in solutions or suspensions. While evaporation yields concentrated liquids or slurries, drying produces solid end products with minimal moisture content.

PURPOSE OF DRYING

Manufacturing Requirements

Pharmaceutical manufacturing extensively utilizes drying operations in various processes, particularly in granulation. This critical step enables efficient downstream processing, including bulk packaging, tablet compression, and capsule filling operations. The process proves indispensable for specialized materials such as aluminum hydroxide and spray-dried excipients like lactose. The precision and control required in pharmaceutical drying operations distinguish them from other industrial drying applications, as product quality and consistency are paramount.

Economic and Processing Benefits

The implementation of drying operations delivers multiple strategic advantages in pharmaceutical processing. Through bulk weight reduction, companies achieve significant savings in transportation and storage costs. The process enhances material friability, particularly beneficial for natural drug processing, facilitating subsequent size reduction operations. Drying serves as a crucial preservation method for animal and vegetable-derived pharmaceuticals, preventing mold growth and degradation. Furthermore, many pharmaceutical compounds, including effervescent salts, aspirin, and antibiotics, demonstrate superior stability in their dried state, extending their shelf life and maintaining therapeutic efficacy.

Moisture Content Assessment

Technical Parameters

Moisture quantification in pharmaceutical materials relies on two primary measurements. Moisture Content (MC) represents the fundamental ratio of moisture weight to total material weight, providing a direct measure of residual moisture. Loss on Drying (LOD) indicates the percentage of moisture lost during standardized drying conditions, serving as a quality control parameter. These measurements are essential for process control and final product specifications, ensuring consistent product quality across batches.

Theoretical Framework of Drying Operations

Initial Adjustment Phase

The preliminary stage of drying involves complex heat and mass transfer phenomena. As the wet material enters the drying environment, it undergoes concurrent heating and evaporative cooling processes. The material temperature gradually increases while surface moisture evaporates, eventually reaching equilibrium at the wet-bulb temperature of the drying air. This dynamic balance establishes the foundation for efficient moisture removal in subsequent phases, determining the overall drying efficiency.

Constant Rate Period

During this critical phase, the material maintains a continuous liquid film on its surface, enabling steady-state evaporation at wet-bulb temperature. The drying rate remains constant as internal moisture continuously migrates to replenish surface evaporation. This period represents optimal drying conditions, where heat and mass transfer rates achieve maximum efficiency. The drying rate correlates directly with factors including surface area, temperature differential, material density, bed thickness, and heat transfer coefficients.

First Falling Rate Period

The transition to the first falling rate period occurs at the critical moisture content (CMC), marking a significant change in drying dynamics. As dry spots emerge on the material surface, both heat and mass transfer rates begin declining. The material temperature increases toward the dry-bulb temperature, while the surface area available for evaporation progressively decreases. This phase represents a crucial transition in the drying process, requiring careful monitoring and control.

Second Falling Rate Period

The final drying phase is characterized by empty capillaries and the absence of surface moisture films. Moisture movement proceeds exclusively through diffusion mechanisms, resulting in progressively decreasing drying rates. The material approaches its equilibrium moisture content (EMC), representing the ultimate practical endpoint of the drying process. This phase often determines the final product quality and requires precise control to achieve desired specifications.

Process Control and Optimization

Process Parameters

Successful pharmaceutical drying operations depend on careful control of multiple interrelated parameters. The relationship between dry-bulb and wet-bulb temperatures determines the driving force for moisture removal. Exposed surface area and material bed thickness affect heat and mass transfer rates, while air humidity and flow rates influence drying efficiency. Understanding and controlling these parameters enables consistent product quality and optimal process efficiency.

Drying Curve Analysis

The systematic analysis of drying curves provides valuable insights for process development and optimization. These curves enable accurate estimation of batch drying times and facilitate equipment sizing calculations. Through careful study of drying curves, manufacturers can establish optimal operating parameters and quality control metrics, ensuring consistent product quality while maximizing operational efficiency.

Equilibrium Considerations

The concept of equilibrium moisture content represents a fundamental limitation in drying operations. This parameter varies with material properties and environmental conditions, establishing the practical endpoint for moisture removal. Understanding EMC behavior enables proper process endpoint determination and helps maintain product quality specifications. The relationship between EMC and operating conditions guides process design and control strategies.

Process Engineering Applications

Equipment selection for pharmaceutical drying operations requires careful consideration of production requirements, material characteristics, and energy efficiency. Modern drying systems incorporate sophisticated control systems to maintain optimal conditions throughout the drying cycle. Process optimization focuses on minimizing energy consumption while maintaining product quality and maximizing production rates. These engineering considerations ensure cost-effective operations while meeting stringent pharmaceutical quality standards.

CLASSIFICATION OF DRYERS

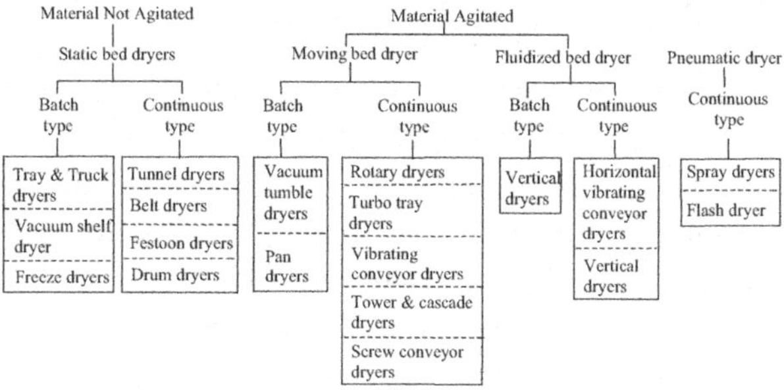

Classification of dryers, based on methods of solids handling

Classification based on heat transfer mechanism

Convection Dryers

Tray/Shelf Dryers

A tray dryer represents one of the most fundamental designs in pharmaceutical drying equipment. The system comprises an insulated cabinet or compartment housing multiple trays containing wet materials. The design incorporates two primary configurations: direct tray placement within the cabinet or a truck system where trays are mounted on wheeled shelves. The trays feature perforated or wire-mesh bottoms to facilitate air circulation. Heat transfer occurs through forced convection, with fans circulating heated air throughout the cabinet while removing moisture-laden air. The heating source typically utilizes either electrical elements or steam systems. This batch-processing equipment proves particularly effective for drying crude drugs, chemicals, powders, and tablet granules, offering the advantage of separate material handling capabilities.

Rotary Dryers

The rotary dryer consists of a long cylindrical shell, typically extending ten meters, mounted at a slight incline. The shell rotates slowly at approximately 10 revolutions per minute, with internal baffles or flights that lift and cascade materials through the airstream. This continuous tumbling action, combined with counter-current hot air flow, ensures efficient heat and mass transfer. The design excels in continuous, large-scale drying operations for powdered or granular pharmaceutical solids, providing consistent product quality through uniform exposure to drying conditions.

Fluidized Bed Dryers

Fluidized bed technology represents an advanced drying system operating on the principle of particle suspension in an upward-flowing air stream. The system progresses through distinct phases as air velocity increases: initial static bed, minimum fluidization, particle rearrangement, full fluidization, and eventual entrainment. The equipment comprises several key components: an air handler for supplying conditioned air, a plenum for air distribution, a product container, an expansion chamber for particle suspension, and filtration systems for fine particle collection.

Conduction Dryers

Vacuum Dryers

Vacuum drying technology utilizes conductive heat transfer under reduced pressure conditions. The system consists of a jacketed vessel with integrated shelf supports for enhanced heat conduction. The chamber connects to a vacuum pump through a condenser and receiver system. This configuration offers several advantages: low-temperature drying capability for thermolabile materials, minimized oxidation risk, production of porous products, and solvent recovery possibilities. However, the reduced heat transfer coefficients result in slower drying rates and higher operational costs.

Freeze Dryers

Freeze drying, or lyophilization, represents a specialized drying process combining vacuum technology with sublimation principles. The process involves freezing the product followed by primary drying (sublimation) and secondary drying (desorption) under vacuum conditions. This technology proves essential for preserving sensitive biological materials and producing highly stable pharmaceutical products.

Radiant Heat Dryers

Infrared Dryers

Infrared drying technology employs electromagnetic radiation for heat transfer, typically in the infrared spectrum. The system directs radiant energy toward the product surface, causing molecular vibration and subsequent moisture removal. This method offers advantages in terms of energy efficiency and precise temperature control, particularly suitable for surface drying applications and heat-sensitive materials.

Each drying technology presents unique advantages and limitations, requiring careful consideration of product characteristics, process requirements, and economic factors in selection and implementation. Understanding these aspects enables pharmaceutical manufacturers to optimize drying operations for specific applications while maintaining product quality and process efficiency

FREEZE DRYER

Operating Principle

The fundamental principle involves operating below the triple point of the solvent to be dried. For water, this point is at 4579 μm Hg and 0.0099°C. Under these conditions, the ice directly sublimes to vapor without passing through the liquid phase. The process typically operates at temperatures between -10°C to -40°C and pressures ranging from 2000 to 100 μm Hg. This enables gentle drying of sensitive pharmaceutical products while maintaining their integrity.

Components

The freeze dryer consists of four essential components. First, a vacuum drying chamber available in both batch and continuous configurations handles the primary drying process. Second, a vacuum source utilizing either a vacuum pump, steam ejector, or a combination of both maintains the required low pressure. Third, a heat source employing either conduction or radiation provides the necessary energy for sublimation. Fourth, a vapor removal system incorporating condensers, desiccants, pumps, or scraper blades efficiently removes the sublimed vapor.

Process Stages

The freeze-drying process begins with preparation and pretreatment, which may include pre-concentration for protein solutions to improve efficiency. During pre-freezing, products are frozen in vials or ampoules using various cooling methods such as cold shelves (-50°C), alcohol baths (-50°C), or liquid nitrogen (-195°C). The optimal freezing rate is maintained between 3-25°C/min, with a target layer thickness of 0.5-0.75 inches.

Primary drying occurs under 0.5 bar vacuum with temperature raised to 30°C, removing 98-99% moisture through sublimation. Secondary drying follows at 0.07 bar vacuum, extending for 10-20 hours to remove residual moisture. The process concludes with packaging, where inert gas is introduced and immediate sealing is performed to maintain product stability.

SPRAY DRYER

Operating Principle

Spray drying involves the transformation of liquid feed into dried particles through atomization and subsequent drying. The process creates small droplets that rapidly dry into solid particles, making it suitable for solutions, suspensions, or pastes.

Components and Process Stages

The atomization systems come in three main varieties. Centrifugal atomizers excel with thermolabile and viscous materials. Pressure atomizers produce coarser particles and are simpler in operation. Pneumatic atomizers offer flexibility in handling various viscosities and produce uniform particles.

The spray-air contact occurs either through co-current flow, ideal for heat-sensitive materials, or counter-current flow, suitable for thermostable materials. The drying mechanism involves surface moisture evaporation and internal moisture migration, with final product characteristics depending on the surface layer properties.

FLASH DRYER

Operating Characteristics

Flash drying employs extremely high-velocity air (300-600 ft/min) at elevated temperatures (300-1300°F) to achieve rapid moisture removal. The process suspends wet solid mass in a finely divided state, creating extensive surface area for efficient drying. Product collection occurs through cyclone separators followed by bag filters or wet scrubbers.

Applications

Freeze drying excels in preserving microbial cultures, antibiotics, blood products, and surgical materials. Spray drying finds extensive use in pharmaceutical processing through standard open cycle, aseptic open cycle, and closed cycle operations. It's particularly valuable for spray congealing, particle coating, taste masking, and sustained release formulations. Flash drying serves best in processing heat-resistant materials where rapid drying and high throughput are essential.

Each drying technology offers unique advantages and limitations, making their selection critical based on specific product requirements, process constraints, and desired final product characteristics. Understanding these differences enables pharmaceutical manufacturers to choose the most appropriate drying method for their specific applications.

Summary

Drying is an essential unit operation in pharmaceutical manufacturing, involving the removal of liquid, typically water, from a solid, semi-solid, or liquid material. This process is crucial for improving product stability, reducing microbial growth, and preparing materials for further processing or storage. Various drying methods are employed in pharmaceutical production, each suited to different materials and end-product requirements. Tray drying, a simple and widely used method, involves spreading the material on trays and exposing it to heated air in a static or circulating system. Fluidized bed drying suspends particles in an upward-flowing air stream, providing rapid and uniform drying. Spray drying atomizes liquid feed into fine droplets that dry quickly in a hot air stream, producing fine powders suitable for inhalation products and improving solubility of poorly water-soluble drugs. Freeze drying (lyophilization) removes water through sublimation under vacuum conditions, preserving the structure of sensitive materials like proteins and vaccines. Vacuum drying operates at reduced pressure, allowing for lower drying temperatures suitable for heat-sensitive compounds. The drying process is governed by heat and mass transfer principles, with factors such as temperature, humidity, air velocity, and material properties influencing drying rates and efficiency. Drying kinetics typically follow a constant rate period followed by a falling rate period, with critical moisture content marking the transition between these phases. Monitoring and control of drying processes often involve measurement of parameters like moisture content, temperature, and airflow. Near-infrared spectroscopy and other PAT tools are increasingly used for real-time monitoring of drying processes. Challenges in pharmaceutical drying include preventing thermal degradation of active ingredients, maintaining desired particle characteristics, and ensuring uniform moisture content throughout the batch. Selection of appropriate drying methods and conditions is crucial to preserve product quality attributes such as particle size, crystal form, and dissolution properties. Energy efficiency and environmental considerations are becoming increasingly important in the design and operation of pharmaceutical drying processes.

Multiple Choice Questions

1. What is the primary purpose of drying in pharmaceutical manufacturing?
   a) To increase particle size
   b) To remove moisture or solvent
   c) To enhance drug stability
   d) To increase bulk density
2. Which of the following is NOT a method of drying?
   a) Tray drying
   b) Freeze drying
   c) Spray drying
   d) Wet granulation
3. The term "bound moisture" refers to:
   a) Water physically adsorbed on the surface
   b) Water chemically bound to the material
   c) Water trapped in pores
   d) Water in the surrounding air
4. Which type of dryer is most suitable for heat-sensitive materials?
   a) Tray dryer
   b) Fluidized bed dryer
   c) Freeze dryer
   d) Spray dryer
5. The principle of sublimation is used in which type of drying?
   a) Tray drying
   b) Freeze drying
   c) Spray drying
   d) Microwave drying
6. Which of the following factors does NOT affect drying rate?
   a) Temperature
   b) Humidity

c) Air velocity
d) Color of the material

7. What is the main advantage of using a fluidized bed dryer?
a) Low energy consumption
b) Uniform drying and high heat transfer
c) Ability to handle wet materials
d) Suitability for thermolabile substances
8. The process of drying where moisture is removed without passing through the liquid state is called:
a) Evaporation
b) Sublimation
c) Condensation
d) Absorption
9. Which type of dryer is most suitable for continuous drying of solutions or suspensions?
a) Tray dryer
b) Freeze dryer
c) Spray dryer
d) Vacuum dryer
10. The term "critical moisture content" in drying refers to:
a) The maximum allowable moisture content
b) The moisture content at which the drying rate changes
c) The initial moisture content of the material
d) The moisture content of the surrounding air
11. Which of the following is an example of a conduction dryer?
a) Spray dryer
b) Fluidized bed dryer
c) Tray dryer
d) Freeze dryer
12. The principle of atomization is used in which type of drying?

a) Tray drying
b) Freeze drying
c) Spray drying
d) Vacuum drying

13. Which type of dryer is most suitable for drying thermolabile materials in bulk?
    a) Tray dryer
    b) Fluidized bed dryer
    c) Vacuum dryer
    d) Spray dryer
14. The term "equilibrium moisture content" refers to:
    a) The initial moisture content of the material
    b) The moisture content at which drying stops under given conditions
    c) The maximum moisture content allowed in the product
    d) The moisture content of the drying air
15. Which of the following factors contributes to increased drying efficiency?
    a) Decreased temperature
    b) Increased humidity
    c) Decreased air velocity
    d) Increased surface area of material

List of Important Questions

1. What is drying, and why is it important in pharmaceutical manufacturing?
2. Describe the different mechanisms of moisture removal during drying.
3. What is the significance of the drying curve in understanding the drying process?
4. How does tray drying work, and what are its applications in pharmaceuticals?
5. Explain the principle of fluidized bed drying and its advantages.
6. What are the key features of spray drying, and when is it preferred?
7. How does freeze drying (lyophilization) differ from other drying methods?
8. Describe the working principle of a rotary dryer and its applications.
9. What are the factors affecting the rate of drying in pharmaceutical processes?
10. How does the glass transition temperature affect the drying of amorphous materials?
11. Explain the concept of equilibrium moisture content and its importance in drying.
12. What are the challenges in drying heat-sensitive pharmaceutical materials?
13. How is the efficiency of a drying process evaluated and optimized?
14. Describe the role of drying in improving the stability of pharmaceutical products.
15. What are the latest innovations in drying technology for pharmaceuticals?

Bibliography

1. Mujumdar AS, editor. Handbook of industrial drying. 4th ed. Boca Raton: CRC Press; 2014.
2. Keey RB. Drying of loose and particulate materials. New York: Hemisphere Publishing Corporation; 1992.
3. Strumillo C, Kudra T. Drying: principles, applications and design. New York: Gordon and Breach Science Publishers; 1986.
4. Chen XD, Mujumdar AS, editors. Drying technologies in food processing. Oxford: Blackwell Publishing; 2008.
5. Oakley DE. Produce uniform particles by spray drying. Chem Eng Prog. 1997;93(10):48-54.
6. Kudra T, Mujumdar AS. Advanced drying technologies. 2nd ed. Boca Raton: CRC Press; 2009.
7. Van't Land CM. Industrial drying equipment: selection and application. New York: Marcel Dekker; 1991.
8. Delgado JMPQ, Barbosa de Lima AG, editors. Drying and energy technologies. Cham: Springer; 2016.
9. Mujumdar AS, editor. Drying '92. Amsterdam: Elsevier; 1992.
10. Arun S. Mujumdar, editor. Handbook of industrial drying. 3rd ed. Boca Raton: CRC Press; 2006.

CHAPTER 10

EXTRACTION

Author

Mrs. Swarupa Ameya Salvi

Assistant Professor, Department of Chemistry, Sathaye College, Mumbai, Maharashtra, India

Abstract

Extraction is a fundamental separation process in pharmaceutical manufacturing, used to isolate desired compounds from natural sources or to purify synthetic products. This technique relies on the principle of differential solubility, where the target compound preferentially dissolves in a selected solvent. Various extraction methods are employed, including liquid-liquid extraction, solid-liquid extraction, and supercritical fluid extraction, each suited to different types of raw materials and target compounds. Factors influencing extraction efficiency include solvent choice, temperature, pH, and contact time. The concept of partition coefficient is explored to understand the distribution of compounds between immiscible phases. Advanced extraction techniques, such as microwave-assisted extraction and ultrasound-assisted extraction, are discussed in the context of improving yield and reducing processing time. Continuous extraction processes, including percolation and Soxhlet extraction, are examined for their applications in large-scale pharmaceutical production. Quality control measures, including assay of extracted compounds and solvent residue testing, are essential to ensure product purity and safety

Keywords: *Solvent extraction, Partition coefficient, Natural product isolation, Purification, Continuous extraction, Process optimization*

Learning Objectives

After completion of the chapter, the student should be able to:

- Define extraction and its applications in pharmaceutical processing.
- Explain the principles and mechanisms of various extraction techniques.
- Describe different types of extraction equipment used in pharmaceuticals.
- Discuss the factors affecting extraction efficiency and yield.
- Explain the concept of solvent selection and its importance in extraction processes.
- Analyze the challenges in extracting different types of pharmaceutical compounds.
- Evaluate methods for optimizing extraction processes in drug development and production.

Extraction stands as a cornerstone process in pharmaceutical manufacturing, playing a vital role in isolating and purifying medicinal compounds. This process, developed over centuries of pharmaceutical practice, has evolved from simple plant extractions to sophisticated industrial-scale operations. In pharmaceutical sciences, extraction serves as the primary method for obtaining pure drug substances from natural sources and purifying synthetic pharmaceutical compounds.

The process of extraction involves separating desired substances from a mixture by using a solvent in which the target compound is soluble while other substances remain insoluble. This selective separation is based on the fundamental principle of differential solubility, where compounds distribute themselves between two immiscible phases according to their solubility characteristics.

asic Principles of Extraction

Differential Solubility

The principle of differential solubility forms the foundation of extraction processes. When a substance encounters two immiscible liquids, it naturally distributes itself between them based on its relative solubility in each phase. This distribution is not random but follows specific physicochemical principles. The degree of solubility in each phase depends on various factors including molecular structure, polarity, temperature, and pH. For instance, in the extraction of alkaloids from plant materials, the addition of acid makes the alkaloids water-soluble by converting them to their salt forms, while subsequent basification allows their extraction into organic solvents.

Mass Transfer

Mass transfer in extraction is a complex phenomenon that occurs at the interface between phases. During the extraction process, molecules of the desired compound move from one phase to another until equilibrium is established. This transfer is governed by concentration gradients and interfacial phenomena. The efficiency of mass transfer depends significantly on the surface area of contact between the phases. Increasing the surface area through proper mixing or agitation enhances the rate of extraction. Temperature also plays a crucial role, as higher temperatures generally increase molecular motion and solubility, leading to faster mass transfer rates. However, temperature must be carefully controlled to prevent degradation of heat-sensitive compounds.

Distribution Law

Nernst's Distribution Law provides the theoretical foundation for understanding how compounds distribute themselves between phases during extraction. The law states that at constant temperature, regardless of the total amount of solute present, the ratio of concentrations between two immiscible phases remains constant. This ratio, known as the distribution coefficient (K), is expressed mathematically as $K = C1/C2$, where C1 and C2 are the equilibrium concentrations in the respective phases. This law helps in predicting the number of extraction steps needed and the efficiency of the extraction process. Understanding the distribution coefficient is crucial for optimizing extraction procedures and maximizing yield.

Applications in Pharmaceutical Processing

Natural Product Isolation

The extraction of medicinal compounds from natural sources remains one of the primary applications in pharmaceutical processing. This field has historically been crucial in drug discovery and continues to be relevant in modern pharmaceutical production. The process begins with the careful selection of plant or animal material, followed by appropriate preparation methods such as drying, grinding, or powdering to maximize extraction efficiency. Different compounds require different extraction approaches - for instance, morphine extraction from opium poppy involves careful pH control and multiple solvent extraction steps, while essential oil extraction might require steam distillation or cold pressing methods. The isolation of quinine from cinchona bark exemplifies how extraction techniques have evolved from traditional methods to modern industrial processes.

Industrial Applications

In modern pharmaceutical manufacturing, extraction processes have become highly sophisticated and are utilized at various stages of drug production. Drug purification through extraction is a critical step in ensuring pharmaceutical quality. After chemical synthesis, crude drug products often contain impurities that must be removed through carefully designed extraction procedures. These processes require precise control of parameters such as solvent selection, pH, temperature, and mixing conditions.

EXTRACTION TECHNIQUES AND METHODOLOGIES

Liquid-Liquid Extraction

Liquid-liquid extraction, also known as solvent extraction, is a fundamental technique in pharmaceutical processing. This method exploits the difference in solubility of compounds between two immiscible liquid phases, typically an aqueous phase and an organic solvent. The process begins with the mixing of these phases, during which the desired compound preferentially moves into the phase where it has higher solubility. The success of liquid-liquid extraction depends heavily on the choice of solvents. Common organic solvents include chloroform, ethyl acetate, and hexane, each selected based on the polarity and chemical properties of the target compound.

The efficiency of liquid-liquid extraction can be enhanced through multiple extractions using smaller volumes of solvent rather than a single extraction with a larger volume. This principle is demonstrated by the equation:

$E = 1 - (Vw/KVo + Vw)n$

Where:

E = Extraction efficiency

Vw = Volume of aqueous phase

Vo = Volume of organic phase

K = Distribution coefficient

n = Number of extractions

Solid-Liquid Extraction

Solid-liquid extraction, or leaching, involves the removal of soluble components from solid materials using suitable solvents. This method is particularly important in the extraction of active compounds from plant materials. The process occurs in several stages: first, the solvent penetrates the solid matrix; second, the compound dissolves in the solvent; and finally, the dissolved compound diffuses out of the solid matrix.

Several factors influence the efficiency of solid-liquid extraction:

Contact Time: Longer contact between solvent and solid material generally increases yield, though this must be balanced against practical considerations and potential degradation of compounds.

Particle Size: Smaller particle sizes increase surface area and improve extraction efficiency, but extremely fine particles may cause problems in subsequent separation steps.

Temperature: Higher temperatures typically improve solubility and diffusion rates, but may lead to thermal degradation of sensitive compounds.

Continuous Extraction Methods

Soxhlet Extraction

The Soxhlet apparatus represents a milestone in extraction technology, providing continuous extraction of solid materials. In this method, fresh solvent repeatedly passes through the solid material, maintaining a concentration gradient that favors continued extraction. The process operates automatically once started, making it highly efficient for complete extraction of compounds from plant materials.

The main components of a Soxhlet extractor include:

- A thimble holder containing the solid material
- A distillation flask for heating the solvent
- A condenser for cooling and recycling the solvent
- A siphon mechanism for automatically emptying the extraction chamber

Percolation

Percolation involves the continuous passage of solvent through a bed of solid material. This method is particularly useful for large-scale pharmaceutical extractions. The process can be modified by varying:

- Flow rate of solvent
- Temperature of extraction
- Pressure applied to the system
- Solvent composition

Modern Extraction Technologies

Supercritical Fluid Extraction

Supercritical fluid extraction (SFE) represents a significant advancement in extraction technology. This method typically uses carbon dioxide in its supercritical state, where it exhibits properties of both gases and liquids. The advantages of SFE include:

Temperature Control: The relatively low critical temperature of CO_2 (31.1°C) allows extraction of heat-sensitive compounds without degradation.
Selectivity: The solvating power can be fine-tuned by adjusting pressure and temperature.
Environmental Impact: CO_2 is environmentally friendly and leaves no toxic residues.

PROCESS OPTIMIZATION AND QUALITY CONTROL

Factors Affecting Extraction Efficiency

Temperature Control

Temperature plays a critical role in extraction processes by influencing both solubility and mass transfer rates. Higher temperatures generally increase the solubility of compounds and reduce solvent viscosity, leading to improved extraction efficiency. However, temperature optimization must consider several factors. For thermolabile compounds, elevated temperatures can cause degradation, necessitating lower temperature operations. The relationship between temperature and extraction efficiency follows the Arrhenius equation, where the rate of extraction typically doubles for every 10°C increase in temperature, up to an optimal point.

pH Management

The pH of the extraction system significantly influences the ionization state of compounds, particularly for alkaloids and organic acids. In alkaloid extraction, pH manipulation is used to convert compounds between their salt and free base forms. At low pH, alkaloids exist as water-soluble salts, while at high pH, they convert to free bases soluble in organic solvents. This principle is utilized in acid-base extraction procedures, where sequential pH adjustments enable selective extraction of different compound classes.

Solvent Selection

The choice of solvent is perhaps the most crucial factor in extraction design. Ideal extraction solvents should possess:

Selectivity: The ability to preferentially dissolve the target compound while leaving unwanted substances behind.

Safety: Low toxicity and environmental impact, considering both operator safety and final product quality.

Physical Properties: Appropriate boiling point, viscosity, and density for efficient separation and recovery.

Common pharmaceutical extraction solvents include:

Water: Used for polar compounds and initial extraction of plant materials.

Ethanol: Excellent for intermediate polarity compounds and generally safe for consumption.

Methylene chloride: Effective for non-polar compounds but requires careful handling.

Hexane: Suitable for highly non-polar compounds like fixed oils.

Quality Control in Extraction Processes

Standardization Parameters

Quality control in pharmaceutical extraction requires monitoring and standardization of several key parameters:

Raw Material Quality

The quality of starting materials significantly impacts extraction efficiency and final product quality. Standards for raw materials include:

Moisture Content: Must be within specified limits to

prevent microbial growth and ensure consistent extraction.
Particle Size Distribution: Should be uniform and appropriate for the extraction method.
Identity Verification: Through organoleptic, microscopic, and chemical testing.

Process Monitoring

Continuous monitoring of extraction parameters ensures consistency and quality:

In-Process Controls

- Regular sampling during extraction
- Monitoring of solvent composition
- Temperature and pressure tracking
- pH verification at critical points

End-Product Testing

- Assay of active compounds
- Residual solvent analysis
- Microbial contamination testing
- Heavy metal analysis

Optimization Strategies

Experimental Design

Systematic optimization of extraction processes often employs Design of Experiments (DoE) methodology. This approach allows simultaneous evaluation of multiple variables and their interactions. Key aspects include:
Factorial Design: Evaluation of multiple factors at different levels to determine optimal conditions.
Response Surface Methodology: Mathematical modeling to predict optimal extraction conditions.
Statistical Analysis: Determination of significant factors and their interactions.

Scale-up Considerations

When moving from laboratory to industrial scale, several factors must be considered:

Equipment Selection

Industrial-scale extraction equipment must maintain the efficiency of laboratory processes while accommodating larger volumes. Considerations include:

- Heat transfer efficiency
- Mixing characteristics
- Material of construction compatibility
- Ease of cleaning and maintenance

Process Parameters

Scale-up requires adjustment of process parameters:

- Solvent-to-feed ratio optimization
- Adjustment of contact time
- Modification of agitation intensity
- Heat transfer calculations

Summary

Extraction is a fundamental separation process in pharmaceutical manufacturing, used to isolate desired compounds from complex mixtures, often plant or animal tissues. This operation relies on the principle of differential solubility, where target compounds are selectively dissolved in a suitable solvent. Various extraction methods are employed, each tailored to specific applications and compound properties. Solid-liquid extraction, commonly used for plant materials, involves leaching soluble components from a solid matrix. Liquid-liquid extraction separates compounds between two immiscible liquid phases based on their partition coefficients. Supercritical fluid extraction, often using carbon dioxide, offers advantages in extracting heat-sensitive compounds. Factors influencing extraction efficiency include solvent choice, temperature, pH, particle size of the solid material, and contact time. Continuous extraction methods, such as percolation and Soxhlet extraction, enhance yield and reduce processing time. Modern extraction techniques like microwave-assisted extraction and ultrasound-assisted extraction provide rapid extraction with reduced solvent consumption. The choice of extraction method depends on the nature of the target compound, the source material, and the desired end-product characteristics. Solvent selection is critical, considering factors such as selectivity, safety, and environmental impact. Green extraction methods, using eco-friendly solvents and processes, are gaining prominence in pharmaceutical manufacturing. Post-extraction processing often involves concentration, purification, and standardization steps to obtain the final extract. Quality control of extracts includes assays for active constituents, evaluation of physicochemical properties, and testing for residual solvents. Extraction is crucial in the production of many herbal medicines, nutraceuticals, and as a preliminary step in the isolation of active pharmaceutical ingredients from natural sources.

Multiple Choice Questions

1. What is the primary purpose of extraction in pharmaceutical manufacturing?
   a) To increase particle size
   b) To separate desired components from a mixture
   c) To reduce moisture content
   d) To increase bulk density
2. Which of the following is NOT a type of extraction?
   a) Liquid-liquid extraction
   b) Solid-liquid extraction
   c) Supercritical fluid extraction
   d) Particle size extraction
3. The term "partition coefficient" in extraction refers to:
   a) The ratio of solute concentrations in two immiscible phases
   b) The total amount of solute extracted
   c) The time required for complete extraction
   d) The volume of solvent used
4. Which type of extraction is most suitable for heat-sensitive compounds?
   a) Hot continuous extraction
   b) Cold maceration
   c) Soxhlet extraction
   d) Reflux extraction
5. The principle of countercurrent flow is used in which type of extraction?
   a) Simple maceration
   b) Percolation
   c) Multistage extraction
   d) Single-stage extraction
6. Which of the following factors does NOT affect extraction efficiency?

a) Temperature
b) Solvent choice
c) Extraction time
d) Color of the extract

7. What is the main advantage of using supercritical fluid extraction?
   a) Low cost
   b) Simple equipment design
   c) Environmentally friendly and residue-free extracts
   d) Ability to extract all types of compounds
8. The process of extraction where a solid material is contacted with fresh portions of the same solvent is called:
   a) Continuous extraction
   b) Batch extraction
   c) Multistage extraction
   d) Single-stage extraction
9. Which type of extraction is most suitable for extracting volatile oils from plant materials?
   a) Maceration
   b) Percolation
   c) Steam distillation
   d) Soxhlet extraction
10. The term "miscella" in extraction refers to:
    a) The solid residue after extraction
    b) The solution of the extracted substance in the solvent
    c) The equipment used for extraction
    d) The interface between two immiscible liquids
11. Which of the following is an example of a continuous extraction method?
    a) Maceration
    b) Percolation

c) Soxhlet extraction
d) Infusion

12. The principle of diffusion is primarily responsible for which stage of extraction?
a) Solvent selection
b) Mass transfer of solute from solid to liquid
c) Separation of extract from residue
d) Solvent recovery
13. Which type of extraction is most suitable for extracting thermolabile compounds from plant materials?
a) Hot continuous extraction
b) Cold maceration
c) Microwave-assisted extraction
d) Ultrasound-assisted extraction
14. The term "marc" in extraction refers to:
a) The liquid extract
b) The solid residue after extraction
c) The solvent used for extraction
d) The equipment used for extraction
15. Which of the following factors contributes to increased extraction efficiency?
a) Decreased temperature (for non-volatile compounds)
b) Increased particle size of the solid
c) Decreased extraction time
d) Increased solvent polarity (for polar compounds)
16. What is the primary purpose of using a Soxhlet extractor?
a) To perform single-stage extraction
b) To perform continuous extraction with solvent recycling
c) To extract volatile compounds
d) To perform extraction at high pressures

17. The process of extraction where a solid material is continuously washed with fresh solvent is called:
    a) Maceration
    b) Percolation
    c) Reflux extraction
    d) Infusion
18. Which type of extraction is most suitable for extracting large quantities of material in industrial settings?
    a) Soxhlet extraction
    b) Maceration
    c) Percolation in large columns
    d) Infusion
19. The term "menstruum" in extraction refers to:
    a) The solid material being extracted
    b) The solvent or mixture of solvents used for extraction
    c) The extracted compounds
    d) The equipment used for extraction
20. Which of the following techniques can enhance the efficiency of solid-liquid extraction?
    a) Increasing particle size of the solid
    b) Decreasing the solid-to-solvent ratio
    c) Using ultrasound or microwave assistance
    d) Keeping the mixture stationary

List of Important Questions

1. What is drying, and why is it important in What is extraction, and why is it important in pharmaceutical manufacturing?
2. Describe the different types of extraction processes used in pharmaceuticals.
3. What are the key factors affecting the efficiency of an extraction process?
4. How does liquid-liquid extraction work, and what are its applications?
5. Explain the principle of solid-liquid extraction (leaching) and its use in natural product isolation.
6. What is the role of partition coefficient in liquid-liquid extraction?
7. Describe the working principle of a Soxhlet extractor.
8. How does supercritical fluid extraction differ from conventional extraction methods?
9. What are the advantages and limitations of microwave-assisted extraction?
10. Explain the concept of countercurrent extraction and its benefits.
11. How does the choice of solvent affect the extraction process and product quality?
12. Describe the challenges in scaling up extraction processes in pharmaceutical manufacturing.
13. What are the key considerations in extracting heat-sensitive or oxidation-prone compounds?
14. How is the efficiency of an extraction process evaluated and optimized?
15. What are the latest innovations in extraction technology for pharmaceuticals?

Bibliography

1. Bart HJ, Pilz S. Industrial scale natural products extraction. Weinheim: Wiley-VCH; 2011.
2. Rydberg J, Cox M, Musikas C, Choppin GR, editors. Solvent extraction principles and practice. 2nd ed. New York: Marcel Dekker; 2004.
3. Mukhopadhyay M. Natural extracts using supercritical carbon dioxide. Boca Raton: CRC Press; 2000.
4. Chemat F, Strube J, editors. Green extraction of natural products: theory and practice. Weinheim: Wiley-VCH; 2015.
5. Thornton JD. Science and practice of liquid-liquid extraction. Oxford: Clarendon Press; 1992.
6. Sarker SD, Latif Z, Gray AI, editors. Natural products isolation. 2nd ed. Totowa: Humana Press; 2006.
7. Takeuchi TM, Pereira CG, Braga MEM, Maróstica MR Jr, Leal PF, Meireles MAA. Low-pressure solvent extraction (solid–liquid extraction, microwave assisted, and ultrasound assisted) from condimentary plants. In: Meireles MAA, editor. Extracting bioactive compounds for food products: theory and applications. Boca Raton: CRC Press; 2009. p. 137-218.
8. Reverchon E, De Marco I. Supercritical fluid extraction and fractionation of natural matter. J Supercrit Fluids. 2006;38(2):146-66.
9. Azmir J, Zaidul ISM, Rahman MM, Sharif KM, Mohamed A, Sahena F, et al. Techniques for extraction of bioactive compounds from plant materials: a review. J Food Eng. 2013;117(4):426-36.
10. Luque de Castro MD, Priego-Capote F. Soxhlet extraction: past and present panacea. J Chromatogr A. 2010;1217(16):2383-9.

CHAPTER 11

TABLETS

Author

Miss Golla Venkata Sowmyasree
Assistant Professor, Dept of Pharmaceutics,
Annamacharya College of Pharmacy, Rajampet,
Andhra Pradesh, India

Abstract

Tablets are the most widely used solid dosage form in pharmaceutical practice, offering advantages such as precise dosing, stability, and patient convenience. This section explores the various types of tablets, including immediate-release, modified-release, and orally disintegrating tablets, each designed to meet specific therapeutic needs. The composition of tablets, including active ingredients and excipients such as diluents, binders, disintegrants, and lubricants, is discussed in detail. Tablet manufacturing processes, from wet granulation and dry granulation to direct compression, are examined, highlighting the factors influencing the choice of method. Critical quality attributes of tablets, such as hardness, friability, disintegration time, and dissolution rate, are explored along with their testing methods. The principles of tablet press operation and the impact of compression forces on tablet properties are addressed. Coating processes, including film coating and sugar coating, are discussed in relation to their functional and aesthetic benefits. Common tablet defects, their causes, and remedies are outlined to aid in troubleshooting manufacturing issues

Keywords: *Solid dosage form, Compression, Granulation, Dissolution, Coating, Quality control*

Learning Objectives

After completion of the chapter, the student should be able to:

- Define tablets and explain their advantages as a dosage form.
- Describe the different types of tablets and their specific applications.
- Explain the composition and function of various tablet ingredients.
- Outline the manufacturing processes for different types of tablets.
- Discuss the quality control tests and specifications for tablets.
- Analyze common problems in tablet manufacturing and their solutions.
- Evaluate the factors affecting tablet disintegration, dissolution, and bioavailability.

Tablets represent the most widely used pharmaceutical dosage form, accounting for approximately 70-80% of all pharmaceutical preparations. Their popularity stems from their versatility, stability, and patient acceptability. A tablet is a solid pharmaceutical dosage form containing one or more active ingredients and excipients, typically formed by compression of powders into a solid unit dose.

Historical Development and Significance

The evolution of tablets as a dosage form dates back to the late 19th century, with the first tablet press being patented by William Brockedon in 1843. Modern tablet technology has advanced significantly, incorporating sophisticated formulation techniques and manufacturing processes to ensure optimal therapeutic outcomes.

Types of Tablets

Oral Tablets for Ingestion

Table 1: Classification of Oral Tablets

Type	Description	Examples
Immediate Release	Designed to disintegrate and release drug rapidly	Paracetamol tablets
Modified Release	Controls drug release over time	Extended-release metformin
Sublingual	Dissolves under the tongue	Nitroglycerin tablets
Buccal	Adheres to cheek mucosa	Buprenorphine
Chewable	Meant to be chewed before swallowing	Antacid tablets

Tablets Used in Oral Cavity

a) Buccal and Sublingual Tablets

These tablets are designed to release medication for local or systemic effects through the oral mucosa. They bypass first-pass metabolism, offering improved bioavailability for certain drugs.

b) Lozenges

Medicated confections designed to dissolve slowly in the mouth, primarily used for local effects in the throat and oral cavity.

3.Tablets Administered by Other Routes

a) Vaginal Tablets

Specially formulated tablets for insertion into the vaginal cavity, often containing hormones or anti-infective agents.

b) Implantation Tablets

Sterile tablets designed for subcutaneous implantation, providing long-term drug release.

Composition of Tablets

1. Active Pharmaceutical Ingredient (API)
   The therapeutic ingredient responsible for the intended pharmacological effect. The amount of API determines many aspects of the formulation, including:
   - Choice of excipients
   - Manufacturing process
   - Tablet size and weight
   - Quality control parameters
2. Excipients

Table 2: Essential Tablet Excipients and Their Functions

Excipient Type	**Function**	**Common Examples**
Diluents	Bulk addition	Lactose, MCC
Binders	Hold particles together	PVP, HPMC
Disintegrants	Facilitate tablet break-up	Starch, Croscarmellose
Lubricants	Reduce friction	Magnesium stearate
Glidants	Improve flow	Colloidal silica

Diluents (Fillers)

These materials provide bulk to the formulation, particularly important when the drug dose is small.

Common diluents include:

- Lactose (various grades)
- Microcrystalline cellulose
- Dicalcium phosphate
- Mannitol

Selection criteria for diluents include:

- Compatibility with the API
- Cost-effectiveness
- Flow properties
- Compression characteristics

Binders

These agents provide cohesiveness to powder particles, essential for granulation and tablet strength. Key considerations in binder selection include:

- Required binding capacity
- Moisture sensitivity
- Processing method compatibility
- Cost and availability

Manufacturing Processes

Wet Granulation

Wet granulation remains the most widely used method of tablet preparation, particularly suitable for drugs with poor flow properties or compression characteristics.

Process Steps:

a) Mixing of API and excipients
b) Preparation and addition of binding solution
c) Wet massing and granulation
d) Drying of granules (typically to 1-2% moisture content)
e) Sizing of dried granules
f) Blending with external phase
g) Compression

Advantages:

- Improved flow properties
- Better content uniformity
- Enhanced compressibility
- Reduced dust generation

Disadvantages

- Time and energy intensive
- Multiple processing steps
- Potential moisture sensitivity issues
- Higher production costs

2. Dry Granulation

Table 3: Comparison of Granulation Methods

Parameter	**Wet Granulation**	**Dry Granulation**	**Direct Compression**
Process Steps	6-8	4-5	2-3
Equipment Cost	High	Medium	Low
Moisture Sensitivity	Critical	Not Critical	Not Critical
Energy Requirements	High	Medium	Low
Production	Long	Medium	Short

main approaches:

ce

- Feed rate
- Roll speed

Direct Compression

The simplest method of tablet manufacture, suitable for materials with good flow and compression properties.
Requirements for Direct Compression:

- Excellent powder flow
- Good compressibility
- Adequate dilution potential
- Cost-effective

Manufacturing Equipment

Tablet Compression Machines

Table 4: Types of Tablet Presses

Type	Output Rate (tablets/hour)	Advantages	Applications
Single Punch	3,000-6,000	Simple, economical	R&D, small batches
Rotary (10 stations)	60,000-100,000	Medium output	Pilot scale
High-speed rotary	200,000-1,000,000	High productivity	Large scale production

Components of a Tablet Press:

- Hopper system
- Feed frame
- Dies and punches
- Compression wheels
- Ejection system
- Collection system

2. Critical Process Parameters

Compression Force:

- Typically 4-20 kN
- Monitored through:
    - Tablet hardness
    - Thickness
    - Dissolution profile

Speed of Operation:

- Turret speed
- Feeder speed
- Precompression force
- Main compression force

Quality Control Parameters

Physical Parameters

Table 5: Quality Control Tests and Specifications

Test	**Typical Specification**	**Method**
Weight Variation	±5% for >250mg	USP/BP
Hardness	4-10 kg/cm^2	Hardness tester
Friability	<1% weight loss	Friabilator
Disintegration	15 min (immediate release)	Disintegration apparatus

2. Chemical Parameters

Content Uniformity:

- Acceptance Value (AV) ≤15
- Individual values: 85-115%

Dissolution Testing:

- Apparatus selection (USP I-IV)
- Medium selection
- Sampling times
- Acceptance criteria

3. Stability Testing

Storage Conditions:

- 25°C/60% RH (long term)
- 40°C/75% RH (accelerated)

Parameters Monitored:

- Physical appearance
- Assay
- Dissolution
- Degradation products
- Moisture content

Common Tablet Defects and Remedies

Table 6: Troubleshooting Guide

Defect	**Possible Causes**	**Remedies**
Capping	High compression force	Reduce compression force
	Poor moisture content	Adjust granulation moisture
Picking	Sticky granules	Modify binder concentration
Mottling	Poor mixing	Increase mixing time
Lamination	Air entrapment	Add deaeration step

.

Summary

Tablets are the most widely used solid dosage form in pharmaceutical practice, offering advantages in terms of precision of dosing, stability, and patient convenience. The manufacturing process of tablets involves several stages, each critical to the final product quality. Formulation development begins with the selection of excipients, including diluents, binders, disintegrants, and lubricants, each serving specific functions in the tablet. Granulation, either wet or dry, is often employed to improve flow properties and content uniformity of the powder blend. Direct compression, suitable for materials with good flow and compressibility, bypasses the granulation step. The compression process involves filling the die cavity with the powder blend and applying pressure to form the tablet. Tablet presses range from single-station eccentric presses to high-speed rotary presses capable of producing thousands of tablets per minute. Post-compression processes may include coating, which can serve functional (modified release, enteric protection) or aesthetic purposes. Various types of tablets are produced, including immediate-release, modified-release, sublingual, and effervescent tablets, each designed for specific therapeutic needs. Quality control of tablets involves a range of tests including weight variation, hardness, friability, disintegration, and dissolution. Content uniformity testing ensures consistent distribution of the active ingredient throughout the batch. Stability studies are conducted to determine appropriate packaging and shelf life. Challenges in tablet manufacturing include ensuring consistent weight and content uniformity, optimizing disintegration and dissolution profiles, and addressing issues like capping and lamination. Process analytical technology (PAT) is increasingly used to monitor and control critical process parameters in real-time. The development of novel tablet designs, such as orally disintegrating tablets and multi-layer tablets, continues to expand the versatility of this dosage form. Tablets remain a cornerstone of pharmaceutical delivery, balancing efficacy, stability, and patient compliance.

Multiple Choice Questions

1. What is the primary advantage of tablet dosage forms?
   a) Ease of administration
   b) Precise dosing
   c) Stability
   d) All of the above
2. Which of the following is NOT a method of tablet manufacture?
   a) Direct compression
   b) Wet granulation
   c) Dry granulation
   d) Spray coating
3. The term "friability" in tablet testing refers to:
   a) Tablet hardness
   b) Tablet disintegration time
   c) Tablet weight variation
   d) Tablet resistance to abrasion
4. Which excipient is primarily used as a binder in tablet formulation?
   a) Magnesium stearate
   b) Microcrystalline cellulose
   c) Povidone (PVP)
   d) Talc
5. The process of forming larger particles from fine powders in tablet manufacture is called:
   a) Compression

b) Granulation
c) Lubrication
d) Disintegration

6. Which of the following factors does NOT affect tablet disintegration?
a) Binder concentration
b) Compression force
c) Disintegrant type
d) Tablet color

7. What is the main purpose of adding a lubricant in tablet formulation?
a) To increase tablet hardness
b) To reduce friction during compression and ejection
c) To enhance drug dissolution
d) To improve tablet appearance

8. Which type of tablet is designed to release the drug slowly over an extended period?
a) Chewable tablet
b) Sublingual tablet
c) Enteric-coated tablet
d) Extended-release tablet

9. The term "capping" in tablet defects refers to:
a) Partial or complete separation of the top or bottom of the tablet
b) Embedded surface spots on the tablet
c) Breakage of the tablet edges
d) Rough tablet surface

10. Which of the following tests is used to evaluate the uniformity of drug content in tablets?
a) Friability test
b) Hardness test
c) Content uniformity test
d) Disintegration test

11. What is the primary purpose of adding a disintegrant to a tablet formulation?
    a) To increase tablet hardness
    b) To facilitate tablet breakup in the gastrointestinal tract
    c) To improve tablet appearance
    d) To reduce friction during compression
12. Which of the following is an example of a direct compression excipient?
    a) Starch
    b) Lactose monohydrate
    c) Microcrystalline cellulose
    d) All of the above
13. The term "punch" in tablet manufacturing refers to:
    a) The lower part of the die cavity
    b) The upper part of the die cavity
    c) The tool that compresses the powder into a tablet
    d) The device that measures tablet hardness
14. Which type of tablet coating is used to protect the drug from stomach acid?
    a) Sugar coating
    b) Film coating
    c) Enteric coating
    d) Compression coating
15. What is the primary purpose of the pre-compression step in tableting?
    a) To increase tablet hardness
    b) To reduce air entrapment
    c) To improve powder flow
    d) To enhance drug dissolution
16. Which of the following is NOT a common tablet shape?
    a) Round

b) Oval
c) Triangular
d) Caplet

17. The term "weight variation" in tablet testing refers to:
    a) The difference in weight between individual tablets
    b) The total weight of all tablets in a batch
    c) The weight of the tablet coating
    d) The weight of the active ingredient in each tablet
18. Which of the following factors can contribute to tablet lamination?
    a) Excessive lubrication
    b) Air entrapment during compression
    c) Improper granulation
    d) All of the above
19. What is the primary purpose of adding a glidant to a tablet formulation?
    a) To increase tablet hardness
    b) To improve powder flow
    c) To enhance drug dissolution
    d) To reduce friction during compression
20. Which type of tablet is designed to dissolve in the mouth without chewing?
    a) Chewable tablet
    b) Orally disintegrating tablet
    c) Enteric-coated tablet
    d) Buccal tablet.

List of Important Questions

1. What are tablets, and what are their advantages as a dosage form?
2. Describe the different types of tablets used in pharmaceutical formulations.
3. What are the key ingredients in tablet formulations and their functions?
4. How does direct compression differ from wet granulation in tablet manufacturing?
5. Explain the importance of powder flow properties in tablet production.
6. What are the common problems encountered in tablet manufacturing and how are they addressed?
7. Describe the different types of tablet coatings and their purposes.
8. How is tablet hardness measured, and why is it important?
9. What is friability, and how does it affect tablet quality?
10. Explain the concept of disintegration time and its significance in tablet formulation.
11. How does controlled-release technology work in tablet formulations?
12. Describe the process of tablet compression and the factors affecting it.
13. What are the quality control tests performed on tablets?
14. How do excipients affect the bioavailability of drugs in tablet formulations?
15. What are the latest innovations in tablet technology for improving patient compliance?

Bibliography

1. Augsburger LL, Hoag SW, editors. Pharmaceutical dosage forms: tablets. 3rd ed. New York: Informa Healthcare; 2008.
2. Aulton ME, Taylor KMG, editors. Aulton's pharmaceutics: the design and manufacture of medicines. 5th ed. Edinburgh: Elsevier; 2018.
3. Lieberman HA, Lachman L, Schwartz JB, editors. Pharmaceutical dosage forms: tablets. 2nd ed. New York: Marcel Dekker; 1989.
4. Gad SC, editor. Pharmaceutical manufacturing handbook: production and processes. Hoboken: John Wiley & Sons; 2008.
5. Tiwari SB, Rajabi-Siahboomi AR. Extended-release oral drug delivery technologies: monolithic matrix systems. Methods Mol Biol. 2008;437:217-43.
6. Jivraj M, Martini LG, Thomson CM. An overview of the different excipients useful for the direct compression of tablets. Pharm Sci Technolo Today. 2000;3(2):58-63.
7. Alderborn G. Tablets and compaction. In: Aulton ME, editor. Pharmaceutics: the science of dosage form design. 2nd ed. Edinburgh: Churchill Livingstone; 2002. p. 397-440.
8. Banker GS, Anderson NR. Tablets. In: Lachman L, Lieberman HA, Kanig JL, editors. The theory and practice of industrial pharmacy. 3rd ed. Philadelphia: Lea & Febiger; 1986. p. 293-345.
9. Patel S, Kaushal AM, Bansal AK. Compression physics in the formulation development of tablets. Crit Rev Ther Drug Carrier Syst. 2006;23(1):1-65.
10. Armstrong NA. Tablet manufacture. In: Swarbrick J,. Encyclopedia of pharmaceutical technology. 3rd ed. New York: Informa Healthcare; 2007. p. 3653-72.

CHAPTER 12

CAPSULES

Author

Mr. Gourab Saha

Assistant Professor, College of Pharmaceutical Sciences, Berhampur, Ganjam, Odisha, India

Abstract

Capsules are versatile solid dosage forms that offer unique advantages in drug delivery and patient acceptance. This section covers both hard and soft gelatin capsules, exploring their composition, manufacturing processes, and applications. The properties of gelatin and alternative shell materials, including vegetable-based and hydroxypropyl methylcellulose (HPMC) capsules, are discussed in relation to their impact on drug stability and release. Capsule filling processes for powders, granules, pellets, and liquids are examined, including manual, semi-automatic, and fully automatic filling methods. The formulation considerations for capsule contents, including powder flow properties and compatibility with shell materials, are addressed. Modified-release capsule technologies, such as multi-particulate systems and liquid-filled hard gelatin capsules, are explored for their role in controlled drug delivery. Quality control tests specific to capsules, including weight variation, disintegration, dissolution, and content uniformity, are outlined. Common capsule defects, their causes, and prevention strategies are discussed to ensure product quality. The advantages of capsules in terms of taste masking, ease of swallowing, and potential for combination products are highlighted.

Keywords: *Gelatin, Encapsulation, Fill material, Dissclutior, Modified release, Quality control*

Learning Objectives

After completion of the chapter, the student should be

able to:

- Define capsules and compare their advantages to other dosage forms.
- Describe the different types of capsules (hard and soft) and their applications.
- Explain the composition and properties of capsule shell materials.
- Outline the manufacturing processes for hard and soft gelatin capsules.
- Discuss the quality control tests and specifications for capsules.
- Analyze the factors affecting capsule stability and dissolution.
- Evaluate the role of capsules in modified release drug delivery systems.

Capsules represent a significant advancement in pharmaceutical dosage forms, offering unique advantages in drug delivery and patient compliance. The word "capsule" derives from the Latin "capsula," meaning small box or container.

Types of Capsules

Table 1: Basic Classification of Capsules

Type	**Characteristics**	**Common Applications**
Hard Gelatin	Two-piece shell	Powder/granule fills
Soft Gelatin	One-piece shell	Liquid/semi-solid fills
HPMC	Vegetarian alternative	Moisture-sensitive drugs
Pullulan	Natural polymer	Specialized applications

Hard Gelatin Capsules

Structure and Components:

- Cap and body design
- Standard sizes (000 to 5)
- Lock-ring mechanism
- Various colors available

Advantages:

- Taste masking
- Easy to swallow
- Versatile filling options
- Product identification

2. Soft Gelatin Capsules

Characteristics:

- One-piece construction
- Hermetically sealed
- Variable shapes possible
- Higher moisture content

Shell Composition and Properties

Gelatin-Based Shells

Table 2: Gelatin Types and Properties

Property	**Type A Gelatin**	**Type B Gelatin**
Source	Porcine skin	Bovine hide
Isoelectric point	7-9	4.8-5.2
Bloom strength	150-280	150-280
Viscosity	Variable	Variable

Components:

- Gelatin (12-15%)
- Plasticizers (20-30%)
- Water (13-16%)
- Colorants/Opacifiers

2. Alternative Shell Materials

HPMC Capsules:

- Vegetarian source

- Lower moisture content
- Better stability
- pH independent

Manufacturing Processes

Hard Gelatin Capsule Production

Table 3: Manufacturing Steps

Step	Process	Critical Parameters
Dipping	Pin immersion	Temperature control
Drying	Controlled environment	Humidity/airflow
Trimming	Mechanical cutting	Precision/alignment
Joining	Cap and body assembly	Fit tolerance

Soft Gelatin Capsule Production

Rotary Die Process:
a) Gelatin ribbon formation
b) Fill material insertion
c) Capsule sealing
d) Shape forming
e) Drying and conditioning

Filling Operations

Hard Capsule Filling Methods

Table 4: Filling Equipment Comparison

Method	Output Rate	Accuracy	Application
Manual	Low	Variable	Small scale
Semi-automatic	Medium	Good	Medium scale
Automatic	High	Excellent	Large scale

Fill Material Requirements:

- Appropriate flow properties
- Uniform particle size
- Suitable density
- Moisture content control

2. Fill Material Types

Table 5: Common Fill Materials

Type	Examples	Special Considerations
Powders	APIs, excipients	Flow properties
Pellets	Multiparticulates	Size uniformity
Liquids	Oils, solutions	Compatibility
Semi-solids	Pastes, suspensions	Viscosity control

Quality Control Tests

Physical Tests

Table 6: Quality Parameters and Specifications

Test	Acceptance Criteria	Method
Weight variation	±7.5%	USP/BP
Disintegration	15-30 minutes	Pharmacopoeial
Lock length	Size-specific	Physical measurement
Moisture content	13-16%	Loss on drying

Performance Tests

Dissolution Testing:

- Apparatus selection
- Medium composition
- Sampling intervals

- Acceptance criteria

3. Stability Considerations

Storage Conditions:

- Temperature control
- Humidity monitoring
- Light protection
- Package integrity

Common Defects and Remedies

Table 7: Troubleshooting Guide

Defect	Possible Causes	Solutions
Brittleness	Low moisture	Adjust storage RH
Softening	High humidity	Improve packaging
Splitting	Manufacturing defect	Process optimization
Dissolution failure	Crosslinking	Material selection

Advanced Technologies and Special Applications in Capsule Technology

Modified Release Capsule Systems

Table 8: Advanced Release Technologies

Technology	Mechanism	Applications	Examples
SODAS®	Multi-particulate	Pulsatile release	Verapamil ER
CODECAPS®	Colon targeting	IBD drugs	Mesalamine
Liquid OROS®	Osmotic system	Zero-order release	Controlled release formulations
ProClick®	Dual chamber	Incompatible ingredients	Probiotics

Specialized Capsule Technologies

A. Multi-Compartment Capsules

Features:

- Separated chambers
- Different release profiles
- Incompatible ingredient separation

Applications:

- Combination therapy
- Time-release formulations
- Stability enhancement

Table 9: Multi-Compartment Systems

Type	**Design**	**Advantages**	**Applications**
Capsule-in-Capsule	Nested capsules	Dual release	Fixed-dose combinations
Dual Chamber	Side-by-side	Ingredient separation	Probiotics
Triple Chamber	Three compartments	Complex delivery	Multiple APIs

B. Liquid-Filled Hard Gelatin Capsules (LFHC)

Features:

- Enhanced bioavailability
- Better stability
- Precise dosing

Fill Materials:

- Lipid-based systems
- Self-emulsifying systems
- Thermosoftening matrices

3. Smart Capsule Technologies

A. Programmable Release Systems

Features:

- Electronic components
- Controlled release
- Real-time monitoring

Table 10: Smart Capsule Systems

Technology	Function	Applications	Features
IntelliCap®	Remote controlled	Clinical trials	pH/temp sensing
e-Capsule	Time-controlled	Chronotherapy	Wireless control
SmartPill®	Diagnostic	GI monitoring	Data transmission

B. Targeted Delivery Systems

Technologies:

- pH-responsive coating
- Enzyme-triggered release
- Site-specific delivery

4. Novel Shell Materials and Compositions

Table 11: Advanced Shell Materials

Material	Properties	Advantages	Applications
Pullulan	Natural polymer	Oxygen barrier	Oxygen-sensitive drugs
PVA	Synthetic	Low moisture uptake	Moisture-sensitive drugs
Modified HPMC	Semi-synthetic	Enhanced stability	Extended release

5. Specialized Applications

A. Enteric Capsules

Features:

- Acid resistance
- Intestinal release
- Enhanced stability

Applications:

- Acid-labile drugs
- Gastric irritants
- Targeted delivery

B. Inhalation Capsules

Characteristics:

- Powder containment
- Precise dosing
- Device compatibility

Table 12: Special Purpose Capsules

Type	Design Features	Applications	Benefits
DPI Capsules	Piercing zones	Inhalation drugs	Precise dosing
Enteric Capsules	Acid-resistant	GI targeting	Protection
Chewable Capsules	Soft shell	Pediatric use	Compliance

6. Industrial Innovations

A. 3D Printed Capsules

Applications:

- Customized dosing
- Complex release profiles
- Research applications

Features:

- Precision manufacturing
- Design flexibility
- Rapid prototyping

B. Quality Enhancement Technologies

Table 13: Advanced Quality Control Systems

Technology	Purpose	Advantage
Vision systems	Defect detection	100% inspection
NIR scanning	Content uniformity	Non-destructive
Laser drilling	Modified release	Precision control

7. Environmental Considerations

Sustainable Technologies:

- Bio-based materials
- Recyclable components
- Reduced waste

Table 14: Eco-Friendly Innovations

Innovation	Environmental Impact	Application
Plant-based shells	Biodegradable	Standard capsules
Water-based coating	Low VOC	Modified release
Recycled packaging	Waste reduction	Commercial products

8. Therapeutic Applications

A. Specialty Drug Delivery

Applications:

- Probiotics
- Enzymes
- Hormones
- Peptides

B. Combination Products

Features:

- Multiple APIs
- Different release profiles
- Enhanced therapeutic effect.

Summary

Capsules represent a versatile and widely used dosage form in pharmaceuticals, offering advantages in taste masking, ease of swallowing, and protection of sensitive ingredients. Two main types of capsules are prevalent: hard gelatin capsules and soft gelatin capsules. Hard gelatin capsules consist of two pieces - a body and a cap - and are typically filled with powders or granules. Soft gelatin capsules are one-piece shells filled with liquids or semi-solids. The manufacturing process for hard capsules involves preparing the fill material, which may include blending, granulation, or pelletization steps. Filling machines precisely measure and deposit the powder or granules into the capsule body before closing with the cap. Soft capsule production utilizes a continuous process where the shell material and fill are brought together and sealed simultaneously. Gelatin is the traditional material for capsule shells, but alternatives like hypromellose (HPMC) are gaining popularity, especially for vegetarian formulations and moisture-sensitive drugs. Capsule formulation considerations include fill weight, powder flow properties, and compatibility between the fill and the capsule shell. Modified release capsules can be produced by using special polymers in the shell or by encapsulating coated pellets. Quality control for capsules includes tests for weight variation, content uniformity, disintegration, and dissolution. Capsule integrity tests ensure the absence of defects like cracks or pinholes. Stability studies are crucial, particularly considering potential interactions between the fill and the capsule shell. Challenges in capsule manufacturing include ensuring consistent fill weight, preventing cross-linking in gelatin capsules, and maintaining low moisture content for hygroscopic materials. Specialized capsule designs, such as enteric-coated capsules and capsules with built-in tamper-evidence features, continue to expand the applications of this dosage form. Capsules offer flexibility in formulation, allowing for combination products and customized dosing, making them a valuable option in both mass production and personalized medicine.

Multiple Choice Questions

1. What are the two main types of capsules used in pharmaceutical formulations?
   a) Soft gelatin and hard gelatin capsules
   b) Enteric-coated and non-enteric-coated capsules
   c) Immediate-release and extended-release capsules
   d) Vegetarian and non-vegetarian capsules
2. Which of the following is NOT a common material used in capsule shells?
   a) Gelatin
   b) Hydroxypropyl methylcellulose (HPMC)
   c) Starch
   d) Polyethylene glycol (PEG)
3. The term "lock length" in hard gelatin capsules refers to:
   a) The total length of the capsule
   b) The length of the cap that overlaps the body
   c) The length of the capsule body
   d) The thickness of the capsule shell
4. Which type of capsule is most suitable for liquid or semi-solid formulations?
   a) Hard gelatin capsule
   b) Soft gelatin capsule
   c) HPMC capsule
   d) Enteric-coated capsule

5. What is the primary advantage of using capsules over tablets?
   a) Lower production cost
   b) Better taste masking
   c) Easier to swallow
   d) More stable formulation
6. Which of the following factors does NOT affect capsule disintegration?
   a) Shell material
   b) Fill material properties
   c) Capsule size
   d) Capsule color
7. What is the main purpose of adding a lubricant in capsule formulation?
   a) To increase capsule hardness
   b) To improve powder flow during filling
   c) To enhance drug dissolution
   d) To improve capsule appearance
8. Which type of capsule is designed to release the drug in the intestine rather than the stomach?
   a) Soft gelatin capsule
   b) Hard gelatin capsule
   c) Enteric-coated capsule
   d) Extended-release capsule
9. The term "pelliculation" in capsule manufacturing refers to:
   a) The process of forming the capsule shell
   b) The filling of capsules with powder or granules
   c) The sealing of filled capsules
   d) The coating of capsules
10. Which of the following tests is used to evaluate the uniformity of drug content in capsules?

a) Disintegration test
b) Dissolution test
c) Content uniformity test
d) Weight variation test

11. What is the primary purpose of adding a disintegrant to a capsule formulation?
a) To increase capsule hardness
b) To facilitate capsule breakup in the gastrointestinal tract
c) To improve capsule appearance
d) To reduce friction during filling

12. Which of the following is an advantage of soft gelatin capsules over hard gelatin capsules?
a) Easier to manufacture
b) Can encapsulate liquids and semi-solids
c) More stable formulation
d) Lower production cost

13. The term "body" in hard gelatin capsules refers to:
a) The shorter part of the capsule
b) The longer part of the capsule
c) The entire capsule shell
d) The fill material inside the capsule

14. Which type of capsule filling method is most suitable for large-scale production?
a) Manual filling
b) Semi-automatic filling
c) Automatic filling
d) Dosator nozzle filling

15. What is the primary purpose of band sealing in hard gelatin capsules?
a) To improve capsule appearance
b) To prevent capsule tampering
c) To increase capsule hardness
d) To enhance drug dissolution

16. Which of the following is NOT a common capsule size?
    a) Size 0
    b) Size 00
    c) Size 5
    d) Size 10
17. The term "bloom strength" in gelatin capsules refers to:
    a) The hardness of the capsule shell
    b) The gel strength of the gelatin
    c) The disintegration time of the capsule
    d) The dissolution rate of the drug
18. Which of the following factors can contribute to capsule brittleness?
    a) High humidity during storage
    b) Low moisture content in the capsule shell
    c) Excessive plasticizer in the shell formulation
    d) High fill weight
19. What is the primary purpose of adding a glidant to a capsule formulation?
    a) To increase capsule hardness
    b) To improve powder flow during filling
    c) To enhance drug dissolution
    d) To reduce friction during capsule manufacturing
20. Which type of capsule is designed to float in the stomach for extended drug release?
    a) Enteric-coated capsule
    b) Floating capsule
    c) Time-release capsule
    d) Buccal capsule.

List of Important Questions

1. What are capsules, and what are their advantages as a dosage form?
2. Describe the different types of capsules used in pharmaceutical formulations.
3. What are the main components of hard gelatin capsules?
4. How does the manufacturing process of soft gelatin capsules differ from hard gelatin capsules?
5. Explain the importance of capsule size selection in formulation development.
6. What are the common filling materials used in capsules, and how are they selected?
7. Describe the process of capsule filling and the equipment used.
8. How is capsule disintegration tested, and why is it important?
9. What are the factors affecting the stability of capsule formulations?
10. Explain the concept of liquid-filled hard gelatin capsules and their advantages.
11. How do vegetarian capsules differ from gelatin capsules in terms of properties and applications?
12. Describe the quality control tests performed on capsules.
13. What are the challenges in formulating hygroscopic or deliquescent drugs in capsules?
14. How does particle size of the fill material affect capsule performance?
15. What are the latest innovations in capsule technology for improving drug delivery?

Bibliography

1. Jones BE. Capsules, hard. In: Swarbrick J, editor. Encyclopedia of pharmaceutical technology. 3rd ed. New York: Informa Healthcare; 2007. p. 419-26.
2. Augsburger LL. Hard and soft shell capsules. In: Augsburger LL, Hoag SW, editors. Pharmaceutical dosage forms: tablets. 3rd ed. New York: Informa Healthcare; 2008. p. 395-442.
3. Cole ET, Cadé D, Benameur H. Challenges and opportunities in the encapsulation of liquid and semi-solid formulations into capsules for oral administration. Adv Drug Deliv Rev. 2008;60(6):747-56.
4. Podczeck F, Jones BE. Pharmaceutical capsules. 2nd ed. London: Pharmaceutical Press; 2004.
5. Stegemann S. Hard gelatin capsules today - and tomorrow. Capsugel Library. 2002:1-23.
6. Gullapalli RP. Soft gelatin capsules (softgels). J Pharm Sci. 2010;99(10):4107-48.
7. Kapoor VK, Renna J. Capsules, soft. In: Swarbrick J, editor. Encyclopedia of pharmaceutical technology. 3rd ed. New York: Informa Healthcare; 2007. p. 426-44.
8. Marquardt C, Birkmann C, Neuem-Reulen I. Evaluation of a novel multiparticulate extended release capsule (capsule-in-capsule) system. Drug Dev Ind Pharm. 2013;39(10):1499-507.
9. Ogura T, Furuya Y, Matsuura S. HPMC capsules: an alternative to gelatin. Pharm Technol. 1998;22(11):42-50.
10. Cade D, He X. Gelatin alternatives for the production of hard capsules. Drug Dev Deliv. 2010;4(2):36-9.

CHAPTER 13

LIQUID ORAL PREPARATIONS

Author

Mr. Bharatbhusan Sahu

Assistant Professor, Department of Pharmaceutics, Centurion University of Technology and Management, Rayagada, Odisha, India

Abstract

Liquid oral preparations are versatile dosage forms offering advantages in drug administration, especially for patients with swallowing difficulties. This section covers various types of liquid oral formulations, including solutions, suspensions, emulsions, and syrups. The principles of solubility and factors affecting drug dissolution in liquid media are explored. Formulation considerations, such as pH adjustment, use of co-solvents, and addition of preservatives, are discussed to ensure stability and palatability. The preparation methods for different types of liquid oral formulations are outlined, including techniques for achieving uniform dispersion in suspensions and emulsions. Challenges in liquid formulation, such as taste masking and ensuring dose uniformity, are addressed along with potential solutions. The role of excipients, including sweeteners, flavoring agents, and viscosity modifiers, in improving patient acceptability is examined. Quality control measures specific to liquid oral preparations, such as rheological properties, particle size analysis for suspensions, and stability testing, are detailed

Keywords: *Solutions, Suspensions, Emulsions, Solubility, Palatability, Dose uniformity*

Learning Objectives

After completion of the chapter, the student should be able to:

- Classify different types of liquid oral preparations and their uses.
- Explain the formulation principles of solutions, suspensions, and emulsions.
- Describe the role of various excipients in liquid oral preparations.
- Discuss the manufacturing processes for different liquid oral dosage forms.
- Outline the quality control tests and stability considerations for liquid orals.
- Analyze the challenges in formulating and preserving liquid oral preparations.
- Evaluate the factors affecting the bioavailability of drugs in liquid oral forms.

Liquid oral preparations represent one of the oldest and most fundamental dosage forms in pharmaceutical science. These formulations offer distinct advantages in drug delivery, particularly in terms of dosing flexibility and ease of administration. They are especially valuable for pediatric and geriatric patients who may have difficulty swallowing solid dosage forms. Liquid orals provide rapid drug absorption due to the drug being either dissolved or finely dispersed in a liquid medium, eliminating the disintegration step required for solid dosage forms.

The evolution of liquid oral preparations has progressed from simple solutions to sophisticated delivery systems incorporating advanced technologies for enhanced stability, bioavailability, and patient compliance. These preparations can be broadly categorized into solutions, suspensions, emulsions, and syrups, each with specific characteristics and applications in therapeutic delivery

Classification and Basic Concepts

Table 1: Types of Liquid Oral Preparations

Type	Definition	Examples	Key Features
Solutions	True solutions	Elixirs, Syrups	Homogeneous
Suspensions	Dispersed solids	Antacids	Heterogeneous
Emulsions	Dispersed liquids	Oil-in-water	Two-phase system
Syrups	Sugar solutions	Medicated syrups	High viscosity

1. Solutions

Components:

- Active ingredient
- Solvent system
- Co-solvents
- Preservatives
- Flavoring agents

Advantages:

- Rapid absorption
- Uniform dosing
- Better bioavailability
- Easy administration

2. Formulation Considerations

Table 2: Critical Formulation Parameters

Parameter	Importance	Control Methods
pH	Stability/solubility	Buffers
Viscosity	Flow properties	Thickening agents
Solubility	Drug dissolution	Co-solvents
Stability	Shelf life	Preservatives

Excipients in Liquid Formulations

1. Solvents and Co-solvents

Table 3: Common Solvents

Solvent	Purpose	Concentration Range
Water	Primary solvent	30-90%
Propylene glycol	Co-solvent	10-30%
Glycerin	Co-solvent	5-20%
Ethanol	Co-solvent	5-25%

2. Preservative Systems

Antimicrobial Agents:

- Parabens
- Benzoic acid
- Sorbic acid
- Benzalkonium chloride

3. Taste-Masking Agents

Table 4: Taste-Improving Additives

Agent Type	Examples	Usage Level
Sweeteners	Sucrose, Aspartame	0.1-67%
Flavors	Fruit flavors	0.1-2%
Acids	Citric acid	0.1-1%

Suspension Formulations

1. Key Components

Suspending Agents:

- Xanthan gum
- CMC sodium
- Microcrystalline cellulose

Particle Characteristics:

- Size distribution
- Zeta potential
- Settling rate

2. Stability Considerations

Table 5: Suspension Stability Parameters

Parameter	Acceptable Range	Control Method
Sedimentation	<0.8 rate	Proper viscosity
Particle size	<50 microns	Milling
Redispersibility	Complete in <30s	Structured vehicle

Emulsion Technology

1. Types and Components

Table 6: Emulsion Systems

Type	Continuous Phase	Applications
O/W	Water	Most common
W/O	Oil	Special cases
Multiple	Complex	Controlled release

2. Emulsifying Agents

Types:

- Natural surfactants
- Synthetic surfactants
- Polymeric stabilizers

Manufacturing Processes

1. Solution Preparation

Steps:

a) Solvent selection
b) Order of addition
c) Mixing conditions
d) Filtration
e) Packaging

2. Quality Control Parameters

Table 7: Quality Tests

Test	Specification	Method
pH	Formula-specific	pH meter
Viscosity	Formula-specific	Viscometer
Content uniformity	90-110%	Assay
Microbial limits	USP/BP limits	Microbial testing

Stability Considerations

1. Physical Stability

Factors:

- Temperature
- Light
- Container interaction
- Microbial growth

2. Chemical Stability

Table 8: Stability Parameters

Parameter	Test Method	Frequency
Assay	HPLC/UV	0,3,6,12 months
pH	pH meter	Monthly
Color	Visual/instrumental	Monthly
Clarity	Visual/instrumental	Monthly

Special Formulations

1. Pediatric Formulations

Requirements:

- Taste masking
- Appropriate concentration
- Suitable preservatives
- Safe excipients

2. Modified Release Systems

Table 9: Modified Release Technologies

Technology	Mechanism	Applications
Ion-exchange	Resin binding	Sustained release
Complex formation	Drug-polymer	Taste masking
Multiple emulsion	Phase separation	Controlled release

Quality Control and Documentation

1. Critical Tests

Physicochemical Tests:

- pH
- Viscosity

- Density
- Osmolality

Microbiological Tests:

- Total aerobic count
- Specific organisms
- Preservative efficacy

2. Documentation Requirements

Table 10: Documentation Types

Document	Purpose	Frequency
Master Formula	Manufacturing guide	Per product
Batch Record	Production documentation	Per batch
COA	Quality certification	Per batch

Advanced Formulation Technologies and Special Applications

1. Innovative Delivery Systems

Table 11: Advanced Delivery Technologies

Technology	Mechanism	Applications	Advantages
Nanosuspensions	Particle size reduction	Poor solubility drugs	Enhanced bioavailability
Self-emulsifying systems	Spontaneous emulsification	Lipophilic drugs	Improved absorption
Ion-exchange resins	Drug complexation	Sustained release	Taste masking
Microencapsulation	Particle coating	Stability enhancement	Controlled release

2. Smart Formulation Technologies

A. Responsive Systems

Features:

- pH-triggered release
- Temperature-sensitive delivery
- Enzyme-activated systems

Applications:

- Site-specific delivery
- Timed release
- Enhanced absorption

B. Novel Carrier Systems

Table 12: Advanced Carrier Systems

System	**Components**	**Benefits**	**Applications**
Nanoemulsions	Ultra-small droplets	Enhanced stability	Poorly soluble drugs
Microspheres	Polymeric carriers	Controlled release	Extended action
Cubic phases	Lipid systems	Increased bioavailability	Complex molecules

3. Specialized Formulations

A. Pediatric-Specific Technologies

Features:

- Taste-masking matrices
- Age-appropriate preservatives
- Flexible dosing systems

Table 13: Pediatric Formulation Approaches

Approach	**Technology**	**Benefit**
Mini-drops	Precise dosing	Accuracy
Flavor-burst	Palatability enhancement	Compliance
Growth-	Variable concentration	Flexible

Approach	Technology	Benefit
adjusted		dosing

B. Geriatric Formulations

Considerations:

- Swallowing ability
- Drug-excipient interactions
- Simplified administration

4. Bio-Enhanced Systems

Table 14: Bioavailability Enhancement Approaches

Technology	Mechanism	Application
Cyclodextrin complexation	Inclusion complexes	Solubility enhancement
Solid lipid nanoparticles	Lipid carriers	Improved absorption
Mucoadhesive systems	Increased contact time	Enhanced bioavailability

5. Novel Preservation Technologies

A. Natural Preservative Systems

Components:

- Essential oils
- Plant extracts
- Natural antimicrobials

B. Physical Preservation Methods

Table 15: Advanced Preservation Methods

Method	Mechanism	Advantage
Aseptic processing	Sterile filtration	Chemical-free
Modified atmosphere	Gas replacement	Extended shelf life
Multicomponent systems	Synergistic action	Reduced concentrations

6. Stability Enhancement Technologies

A. Advanced Stabilization Systems

Features:

- Antioxidant combinations
- Light protection systems
- pH stabilization

B. Packaging Innovations

Table 16: Modern Packaging Solutions

Technology	Feature	Benefit
Smart bottles	UV protection	Photo-stability
Unit-dose systems	Individual packaging	Preserved integrity
Active packaging	Oxygen scavenging	Extended stability

7. Quality Enhancement Technologies

A. Process Analytical Technology (PAT)

Applications:

- Real-time monitoring
- Quality prediction
- Process optimization

Table 17: PAT Implementation

Parameter	Technology	Benefit
Viscosity	In-line rheometry	Continuous monitoring
Particle size	Dynamic light scattering	Real-time analysis
Content uniformity	NIR spectroscopy	Non-destructive testing

8. Environmental Considerations

A. Green Technologies

Features:

- Biodegradable components
- Reduced energy consumption
- Minimal waste generation

B. Sustainable Practices

Table 18: Sustainability Measures

Approach	Implementation	Impact
Bio-based materials	Natural sources	Environmental friendly
Energy efficiency	Process optimization	Reduced carbon footprint
Waste reduction	Recycling systems	Minimal environmental impact

Summary

Liquid oral preparations encompass a diverse range of formulations designed for oral administration, offering advantages in dosing flexibility and ease of administration, particularly for pediatric and geriatric patients. These preparations include solutions, suspensions, emulsions, and syrups. Solutions contain dissolved active ingredients in a suitable solvent, often water, and may include co-solvents like ethanol or glycerin to improve solubility. Suspensions consist of finely divided insoluble drugs dispersed in a liquid medium, requiring careful formulation to maintain stability and ensure dose uniformity. Emulsions, either oil-in-water or water-in-oil, are used for drugs that are insoluble in aqueous media. Syrups are concentrated sugar solutions that can mask unpleasant tastes and improve palatability. Formulation of liquid orals involves careful selection of excipients, including preservatives to prevent microbial growth, antioxidants to protect against degradation, flavoring agents to enhance palatability, and viscosity modifiers to improve stability and mouth feel. pH adjustment is often critical to ensure drug stability and optimize absorption. Manufacturing processes for liquid orals typically involve mixing, homogenization, and filtration steps. Specialized equipment such as high-shear mixers and homogenizers are used to ensure uniform dispersion of ingredients. Quality control measures include tests for pH, viscosity, specific gravity, and content uniformity. Stability testing is crucial, considering factors like temperature, light exposure, and container interactions. Challenges in liquid oral formulations include maintaining suspension homogeneity, preventing crystal growth in supersaturated solutions, and ensuring dose accuracy with viscous preparations. Packaging considerations are important, with child-resistant closures and dosing devices often required. Novel approaches in liquid oral preparations include the development of taste-masked formulations, controlled-release liquid systems, and the use of nanotechnology to improve drug solubility and bioavailability.

Multiple Choice Questions

1. Which of the following is NOT a type of liquid oral preparation?
   a) Solution
   b) Suspension
   c) Emulsion
   d) Ointment
2. What is the primary advantage of liquid oral preparations over solid dosage forms?
   a) Longer shelf life
   b) Easier to swallow
   c) More accurate dosing
   d) Lower production cost
3. Which of the following excipients is commonly used as a sweetening agent in

liquid oral preparations?
a) Propylene glycol
b) Sorbitol
c) Methylparaben
d) Polysorbate 80

4. The term "flocculation" in suspensions refers to:
a) Particles settling at the bottom
b) Particles forming loose aggregates
c) Particles forming a cake
d) Particles floating on the surface

5. Which type of emulsion has oil as the dispersed phase and water as the continuous phase?
a) Oil-in-water (O/W) emulsion
b) Water-in-oil (W/O) emulsion
c) Multiple emulsion
d) Microemulsion

6. What is the primary purpose of adding a preservative to a liquid oral preparation?
a) To improve taste
b) To prevent microbial growth
c) To increase viscosity
d) To enhance drug absorption

7. Which of the following factors does NOT affect the stability of a suspension?
a) Particle size
b) Viscosity of the dispersion medium
c) Temperature
d) Bottle shape

8. The term "creaming" in emulsions refers to:
a) Formation of a thick layer on top of the emulsion
b) Separation of oil and water phases

c) Increase in emulsion viscosity
d) Formation of a precipitate

9. Which type of liquid oral preparation is most suitable for water-insoluble drugs?
a) Solution
b) Suspension
c) Syrup
d) Elixir

10. What is the primary purpose of adding a buffering agent to a liquid oral preparation?
a) To improve taste
b) To maintain pH stability
c) To increase viscosity
d) To prevent microbial growth

11. Which of the following is an example of a natural emulsifying agent?
a) Acacia
b) Sodium lauryl sulfate
c) Polysorbate 80
d) Propylene glycol

12. The term "caking" in suspensions refers to:
a) Formation of a hard, compact sediment
b) Floating of particles on the surface
c) Formation of loose aggregates
d) Increase in particle size

13. What is the primary purpose of adding a suspending agent to a suspension?
a) To improve taste
b) To increase viscosity and prevent settling
c) To enhance drug absorption
d) To prevent microbial growth

14. Which of the following is NOT a common method for preparing solutions?
a) Simple dissolution
b) Chemical reaction

c) Extraction
d) Fermentation

15. The term "HLB" in emulsifier selection stands for:
a) High-Level Bonding
b) Hydrophilic-Lipophilic Balance
c) Heavy Liquid Base
d) Hydrogen-Linked Bonding
16. Which type of liquid oral preparation is most suitable for masking the bitter taste of drugs?
a) Solution
b) Suspension
c) Syrup
d) Emulsion
17. What is the primary purpose of adding a wetting agent to a suspension?
a) To improve taste
b) To facilitate dispersion of hydrophobic particles
c) To increase viscosity
d) To prevent microbial growth
18. Which of the following factors can contribute to the instability of an emulsion?
a) Particle size reduction
b) Increase in viscosity
c) Temperature fluctuations
d) Addition of an emulsifier
19. The term "flocculated suspension" refers to:
a) A suspension with uniformly dispersed particles
b) A suspension with particles forming loose aggregates
c) A suspension with a hard, compact sediment

d) A suspension with particles floating on the surface

20. Which of the following is an advantage of using a solution over a suspension?
    a) Better taste masking
    b) Higher drug loading capacity
    c) Faster onset of action
    d) Longer shelf life.

List of Important Questions

1. What are liquid oral preparations, and what are their advantages as dosage forms?
2. Describe the different types of liquid oral preparations used in pharmaceuticals.
3. What are the key components of a liquid oral formulation?
4. How do solutions differ from suspensions in terms of formulation and stability?
5. Explain the importance of pH in liquid oral preparations.
6. What are the common preservatives used in liquid oral formulations, and how are they selected?
7. Describe the process of formulating a stable suspension.
8. How is the viscosity of liquid oral preparations controlled, and why is it important?
9. What are the challenges in formulating poorly water-soluble drugs in liquid oral preparations?
10. Explain the concept of flocculation in suspensions and its significance.
11. How do taste-masking techniques work in liquid oral formulations?

12. Describe the quality control tests performed on liquid oral preparations.
13. What are the factors affecting the stability of liquid oral formulations?
14. How does packaging affect the shelf life of liquid oral preparations?
15. What are the latest innovations in liquid oral preparation technology for improving patient compliance?

Bibliography

1. Allen LV Jr, Popovich NG, Ansel HC. Ansel's pharmaceutical dosage forms and drug delivery systems. 9th ed. Philadelphia: Lippincott Williams & Wilkins; 2011.
2. Niazi SK. Handbook of pharmaceutical manufacturing formulations: liquid products. 2nd ed. Boca Raton: CRC Press; 2019.
3. Nash RA. Suspensions. In: Swarbrick J, Boylan JC, editors. Encyclopedia of pharmaceutical technology. New York: Marcel Dekker; 2002. p. 2045-74.
4. Gennaro AR, editor. Remington: the science and practice of pharmacy. 20th ed. Philadelphia: Lippincott Williams & Wilkins; 2000.
5. Billany MR. Suspensions and emulsions. In: Aulton ME, editor. Pharmaceutics: the science of dosage form design. 2nd ed. Edinburgh: Churchill Livingstone; 2002. p. 334-59.
6. Strickley RG. Solubilizing excipients in oral and injectable formulations. Pharm Res. 2004;21(2):201-30.
7. Florence AT, Attwood D. Physicochemical principles of pharmacy. 6th ed. London: Pharmaceutical Press; 2016.

8. Murthy KS, Ghebre-Sellassie I. Current perspectives on the dissolution stability of solid oral dosage forms. J Pharm Sci. 1993;82(2):113-26.
9. Nairn JG. Solutions, emulsions, suspensions and extracts. In: Genaro AR, editor. Remington: the science and practice of pharmacy. 20th ed. Philadelphia: Lippincott Williams & Wilkins; 2000. p. 721-52.
10. Costantinides PP, Scalart JP, Lancaster C, Marcello J, Marks G, Ellens H, et al. Formulation and intestinal absorption enhancement evaluation of water-in-oil microemulsions incorporating medium-chain glycerides. Pharm Res. 1994;11(10):1385-90.

CHAPTER 14

TOPICAL PREPARATIONS

Author

Dr. Ghangale Gauri Dhondibhau
Assistant Professor, Amrutvahini College of Pharmacy, Sangamner, Maharashtra, India

Abstract

Topical preparations are dosage forms designed for application to the skin or mucous membranes, offering localized drug delivery and systemic effects in some cases. This section covers various types of topical formulations, including creams, ointments, gels, and transdermal patches. The structure and barrier properties of the skin are discussed in relation to drug penetration and absorption. Formulation considerations for topical preparations, such as drug solubility, partition coefficient, and vehicle selection, are explored to optimize drug delivery. The role of penetration enhancers and their mechanisms of action are examined. Manufacturing processes for different topical dosage forms are outlined, including emulsification techniques for creams and fusion method for ointments. Rheological properties of semi-solid preparations and their impact on drug release and application are addressed. Quality control tests specific to topical preparations, including viscosity, spreadability, and in vitro release studies, are detailed. Special considerations for sterile ophthalmic preparations and their packaging requirements are discussed

Keywords: *Dermal delivery, Emulsions, Penetration enhancers, Rheology, Transdermal systems, Bioavailability*

Learning Objectives

After completion of the chapter, the student should be able to:

- Define topical preparations and their routes of administration.
- Classify different types of topical dosage forms and their applications.
- Explain the formulation principles of creams, ointments, gels, and patches.
- Describe the role of various excipients in topical preparations.
- Discuss the manufacturing processes for different topical dosage forms.
- Outline the quality control tests and stability considerations for topicals.
- Analyze the factors affecting drug absorption through the skin.

Topical Preparations are pharmaceutical formulations designed for external application to the skin or mucous membranes. These dosage forms serve both local therapeutic effects and, in some cases, systemic drug delivery. The evolution of topical preparations has led to sophisticated delivery systems that enhance drug penetration, maintain stability, and improve patient compliance.

Classification and Basic Concepts

Table 1: Types of Topical Preparations

Type	Base Type	Applications	Examples
Creams	O/W or W/O	Moisturizing, therapeutic	Antifungal creams
Ointments	Oleaginous	Occlusive therapy	Antibiotic ointments

Type	Base Type	Applications	Examples
Gels	Aqueous/Non-aqueous	Non-greasy application	Anti-inflammatory gels
Patches	Matrix/Reservoir	Systemic delivery	Hormone patches

1. Skin Structure and Drug Penetration

A. Anatomical Considerations

Layers:

- Stratum corneum
- Epidermis
- Dermis
- Hypodermis

B. Penetration Pathways

Table 2: Drug Penetration Routes

Route	Mechanism	Suitable Compounds
Transcellular	Through cells	Hydrophilic drugs
Intercellular	Between cells	Lipophilic drugs
Appendageal	Via follicles	Large molecules

2. Formulation Components

A. Base Materials

Table 3: Common Bases

Type	Examples	Properties
Hydrocarbons	Petrolatum	Occlusive
Vegetable oils	Olive oil	Emollient
Synthetic bases	Polyethylene glycols	Water-soluble

B. Active Ingredients

Categories:

- Anti-inflammatory
- Antimicrobial
- Analgesic
- Hormonal

3. Penetration Enhancers

Table 4: Enhancer Categories

Category	**Examples**	**Mechanism**
Solvents	DMSO, Ethanol	Disruption of SC
Surfactants	Tween, SLS	Lipid extraction
Fatty acids	Oleic acid	Fluidization

Advanced Formulation Technologies

1. Novel Delivery Systems

Table 5: Advanced Delivery Systems

System	**Technology**	**Applications**
Nanoparticles	Lipid/Polymeric	Enhanced penetration
Microspheres	Controlled release	Extended action
Liposomes	Phospholipid vesicles	Improved delivery

2. Smart Delivery Systems

Features:

- pH-responsive
- Temperature-sensitive
- Enzyme-activated

3. Manufacturing Processes

A. Cream Preparation

Steps:

- Phase preparation
- Emulsification
- Homogenization
- Cooling

B. Quality Parameters

Table 6: Critical Quality Attributes

Parameter	**Test Method**	**Specification**
Viscosity	Rheometer	Formula-specific
Spreadability	Parallel plate	Formula-specific

Parameter	Test Method	Specification
pH	pH meter	4.5-8.0

4. Specialized Applications

A. Transdermal Systems

Components:

- Drug reservoir
- Rate-controlling membrane
- Adhesive
- Backing layer

Table 7: Patch Technologies

Type	Design	Applications
Matrix	Drug in adhesive	Small molecules
Reservoir	Membrane controlled	Controlled release
Microreservoir	Dispersed system	Enhanced stability

B. Ophthalmic Preparations

Requirements:

- Sterility
- Isotonicity
- Appropriate viscosity
- Preservative system

5. Stability Considerations

Table 8: Stability Parameters

Parameter	Test Method	Frequency
Physical stability	Appearance	Monthly
Chemical stability	Assay	0,3,6,12 months
Microbial quality	USP methods	Batch release

6. Novel Excipients

Table 9: Advanced Excipients

Category	Examples	Function
Phase transition enhancers	Transcutol	Penetration
Polymeric stabilizers	Carbopols	Rheology

Category	Examples	Function
Natural enhancers	Essential oils	Penetration

7. Quality Control

A. Physical Tests

Parameters:

- Spreadability
- Extrudability
- Texture analysis
- Particle size

B. Performance Tests

Table 10: Performance Evaluation

Test	Method	Purpose
In vitro release	Franz cell	Drug release
Penetration	Tape stripping	Skin delivery
Rheology	Viscometry	Flow properties

8. Special Considerations

A. Environmental Factors

Impact on:

- Stability
- Performance
- Storage conditions

B. Packaging Requirements

Table 11: Packaging Systems

Type	Material	Protection
Tubes	Aluminum/Plastic	Light/Moisture
Jars	Glass/Plastic	Product integrity
Airless	Special design	Contamination

9. Future Trends

Emerging Technologies:

- Smart delivery systems
- Biomimetic materials
- 3D printed topicals

- Personalized formulations

Table 12: Emerging Technologies

Technology	**Feature**	**Benefit**
Smart polymers	Response to stimuli	Controlled release
Bioprinting	Custom formulation	Patient-specific
Nanoemulsions	Enhanced penetration	Better efficacy

Summary

Topical preparations are formulated for application to the skin or mucous membranes, designed to deliver drugs locally or systemically. These preparations encompass a wide range of dosage forms including creams, ointments, gels, lotions, and patches. Creams are emulsions, either oil-in-water or water-in-oil, offering a balance between occlusive and moisturizing properties. Ointments are semi-solid preparations with a greasy texture, providing an occlusive effect that can enhance drug penetration. Gels are semi-solid systems using polymeric thickeners to create a three-dimensional network structure. Lotions are less viscous than creams, typically oil-in-water emulsions or solutions. Transdermal patches deliver drugs systemically through the skin, offering controlled release over extended periods. Formulation of topical preparations involves careful selection of the base, considering factors like drug solubility, desired release rate, and skin compatibility. Penetration enhancers may be included to improve drug absorption through the stratum corneum. Preservatives are often necessary, especially in water-containing formulations. Manufacturing processes for topical preparations include mixing, homogenization, and milling steps to ensure uniform drug distribution and appropriate consistency. Specialized equipment like ointment mills and high-shear mixers are commonly used. Quality control tests for topical preparations include assessments of viscosity, spreadability, pH, and content uniformity. In vitro release testing and skin permeation studies are often conducted to evaluate drug release and penetration characteristics. Stability testing considers factors like phase separation in emulsions, crystal growth in suspensions, and rheological changes over time. Challenges in topical formulation include ensuring adequate drug penetration through the skin barrier, maintaining stability in multi-phase systems, and achieving desired aesthetics and sensory properties. Novel approaches in topical drug delivery include the use of nanocarriers, temperature-responsive gels, and bio-adhesive systems to enhance drug targeting and efficacy.

Multiple Choice Questions

1. Which of the following is NOT a type of topical preparation?
   a) Cream
   b) Ointment
   c) Gel
   d) Syrup
2. What is the primary advantage of topical preparations over oral dosage forms?
   a) Higher bioavailability
   b) Localized drug delivery
   c) Longer shelf life
   d) Lower production cost
3. Which of the following bases is commonly used in water-soluble ointments?
   a) Petrolatum

b) Polyethylene glycol (PEG)
c) Mineral oil
d) Beeswax

4. The term "emollient" in topical preparations refers to:
   a) An agent that increases drug penetration
   b) An agent that softens and smooths the skin
   c) An agent that prevents microbial growth
   d) An agent that increases viscosity
5. Which type of topical preparation is characterized by a semisolid consistency and contains dispersed solid particles?
   a) Solution
   b) Emulsion
   c) Suspension
   d) Paste
6. What is the primary purpose of adding a preservative to a topical preparation?
   a) To improve spreadability
   b) To prevent microbial growth
   c) To increase viscosity
   d) To enhance drug penetration
7. Which of the following factors does NOT affect drug penetration through the skin?
   a) Molecular weight of the drug
   b) Particle size of the drug
   c) pH of the formulation
   d) Color of the formulation
8. The term "occlusivity" in topical preparations refers to:
   a) The ability to block pores
   b) The ability to prevent water loss from the skin
   c) The ability to increase drug solubility
   d) The ability to enhance drug penetration

9. Which type of topical preparation is most suitable for oily skin?
   a) Ointment
   b) Cream
   c) Gel
   d) Lotion
10. What is the primary purpose of adding a penetration enhancer to a topical preparation?
    a) To improve spreadability
    b) To increase drug absorption through the skin
    c) To prevent microbial growth
    d) To improve product stability
11. Which of the following is an example of a natural emollient used in topical preparations?
    a) Mineral oil
    b) Propylene glycol
    c) Aloe vera
    d) Sodium lauryl sulfate
12. The term "phase inversion" in creams refers to:
    a) Change from oil-in-water to water-in-oil emulsion
    b) Separation of oil and water phases
    c) Increase in cream viscosity
    d) Formation of a precipitate
13. What is the primary purpose of adding a humectant to a topical preparation?
    a) To improve spreadability
    b) To retain moisture in the skin
    c) To enhance drug penetration
    d) To prevent microbial growth
14. Which of the following is NOT a common method for enhancing drug penetration through the skin?

a) Using penetration enhancers
b) Microneedles
c) Iontophoresis
d) Centrifugation

15. The term "rubs" in topical preparations refers to:
a) Creams with high water content
b) Ointments with counterirritant properties
c) Gels with cooling effects
d) Lotions with exfoliating properties

16. Which type of topical preparation is most suitable for applying medication to hairy areas?
a) Ointment
b) Cream
c) Lotion
d) Paste

17. What is the primary purpose of adding an antioxidant to a topical preparation?
a) To improve spreadability
b) To prevent oxidation of formulation components
c) To increase viscosity
d) To enhance drug penetration

18. Which of the following factors can contribute to the instability of a cream?
a) Low water content
b) High emulsifier concentration
c) Temperature fluctuations
d) Addition of a preservative

19. The term "cold cream" refers to:
a) A cream stored at low temperatures
b) A water-in-oil emulsion that produces a cooling effect
c) A cream containing menthol or camphor

d) An oil-in-water emulsion used as a moisturizer

20. Which of the following is an advantage of using a gel over an ointment?
    a) Higher drug loading capacity
    b) Better occlusive properties
    c) Ease of application and removal
    d) Longer shelf life.

List of Important Questions

1. What are topical preparations, and what are their advantages as dosage forms?
2. Describe the different types of topical preparations used in pharmaceuticals.
3. What are the key factors affecting drug absorption through the skin?
4. How do ointments differ from creams in terms of composition and applications?
5. Explain the importance of vehicle selection in topical formulations.
6. What are the common penetration enhancers used in topical preparations, and how do they work?
7. Describe the process of formulating a stable emulsion-based topical preparation.
8. How is the viscosity of topical preparations controlled, and why is it important?
9. What are the challenges in formulating water-soluble drugs in topical preparations?
10. Explain the concept of occlusion in topical drug delivery and its significance.
11. How do transdermal patches work, and what are their advantages?
12. Describe the quality control tests performed on topical preparations.

13. What are the factors affecting the stability of topical formulations?
14. How does packaging affect the efficacy and shelf life of topical preparations?
15. What are the latest innovations in topical preparation technology for improving drug delivery?

Bibliography

1. Walters KA, Roberts MS, editors. Dermatological and transdermal formulations. New York: Marcel Dekker; 2002.
2. Williams AC. Transdermal and topical drug delivery: from theory to clinical practice. London: Pharmaceutical Press; 2003.
3. Barry BW. Dermatological formulations: percutaneous absorption. New York: Marcel Dekker; 1983.
4. Osborne DW. Review of changes in topical drug product classification. Pharm Technol. 2008;32(10):66-74.
5. Surber C, Smith EW. The mystical effects of dermatological vehicles. Dermatology. 2005;210(2):157-68.
6. Kulkarni VS, Shaw C. Essential chemistry for formulators of semisolid and liquid dosages. Amsterdam: Elsevier; 2016.
7. Junginger HE. Polymeric permeation enhancers. In: Bronaugh RL, Maibach HI, editors. Percutaneous absorption: drugs, cosmetics, mechanisms, methodology. 4th ed. Boca Raton: Taylor & Francis; 2005. p. 233-52.

8. Benson HAE. Transdermal drug delivery: penetration enhancement techniques. Curr Drug Deliv. 2005;2(1):23-33.
9. Mitragotri S. Devices for overcoming biological barriers: the use of physical forces to disrupt the barrier. Adv Drug Deliv Rev. 2013;65(1):100-3.
10. Otto A, du Plessis J, Wiechers JW. Formulation effects of topical emulsions on transdermal and dermal delivery. Int J Cosmet Sci. 2009;31(1):1-19

CHAPTER 15

NASAL AND EAR PREPARATIONS

Author

Dr. Rakshana V

Assistant Professor, Bharath Institute of Higher Education & Research, Chennai, Tamil Nadu, India

Abstract

Nasal and ear preparations are specialized dosage forms designed for local or systemic drug delivery through the nasal cavity and ear canal. This section explores the anatomy and physiology of the nasal and auditory systems, highlighting their unique features for drug administration. Various types of nasal formulations, including solutions, suspensions, and gels, are discussed along with their applications in local treatment and systemic drug delivery. The formulation considerations for nasal preparations, such as tonicity, pH, and viscosity, are examined to ensure efficacy and patient comfort. Ear preparations, including drops, ointments, and suspensions, are explored with emphasis on their specific requirements for safety and efficacy. The challenges in developing nasal and ear formulations, such as limited residence time and potential for irritation, are addressed along with strategies to overcome them. Advanced delivery systems, including nasal sprays and metered-dose inhalers for nasal administration, are discussed. Quality control measures specific to nasal and ear preparations, including sterility testing, particle size analysis, and spray pattern evaluation, are detailed.

Keywords: *Mucosal delivery, Absorption enhancers, Otic formulations, Spray systems, Local therapy, Bioavailability*

Learning Objectives

After completion of the chapter, the student should be able to:

- Describe the anatomy and physiology of the nasal cavity and ear.
- Explain the advantages and limitations of nasal and ear drug delivery.
- Classify different types of nasal and ear preparations.
- Discuss the formulation principles of nasal sprays, drops, and ear drops.
- Outline the manufacturing processes for nasal and ear preparations.
- Describe the quality control tests specific to nasal and ear formulations.
- Analyze the factors affecting drug absorption in nasal and ear preparations.

Nasal and ear preparations represent specialized pharmaceutical formulations designed for administration through the nasal and auditory routes. These dosage forms offer unique advantages for both local and systemic drug delivery, leveraging the distinct anatomical and physiological characteristics of these organs. Understanding these preparations is crucial for effective therapeutic outcomes in treating various nasal and otic conditions.

I. NASAL PREPARATIONS

1. Anatomical and Physiological Considerations

Table 1: Nasal Cavity Features

Structure	Characteristic	Relevance
Epithelium	Highly vascular	Rapid absorption
Mucosa	Large surface area	Enhanced bioavailability
Cilia	Mucociliary clearance	Drug removal

2. Types of Nasal Formulations

A. Basic Classifications

Table 2: Nasal Preparation Types

Type	Form	Applications
Solutions	Drops/Sprays	Decongestants
Gels	Viscous liquids	Allergic rhinitis
Powders	Dry inhalation	Peptide delivery
Suspensions	Dispersed systems	Local action

3. Formulation Considerations

Key Parameters:

- pH (5.5-6.5)
- Tonicity
- Viscosity
- Sterility

Table 3: Critical Formulation Factors

Parameter	Range	Importance
Osmolality	290-320 mOsm/kg	Comfort
Particle size	<10 µm	Absorption
Surface tension	30-34 mN/m	Spread

II. EAR PREPARATIONS

1. Anatomical Considerations

Structure:

- External ear
- Middle ear
- Inner ear

Table 4: Ear Canal Properties

Feature	**Characteristic**	**Impact**
Length	2.5 cm	Volume limitation
pH	6-7.8	Formulation pH
Surface	Cerumen presence	Drug absorption

2. Types of Ear Preparations

Table 5: Otic Formulation Types

Type	**Properties**	**Uses**
Drops	Aqueous/Oily	Infections
Ointments	Semi-solid	Protection
Suspensions	Dispersed drug	Extended action

Advanced Formulation Technologies

1. Nasal Drug Delivery Systems

A. Novel Carriers

Table 6: Advanced Delivery Systems

System	**Technology**	**Advantage**
Microspheres	Polymeric	Controlled release
Liposomes	Lipid vesicles	Enhanced penetration
Nanoparticles	Colloidal carriers	Improved absorption

2. Smart Delivery Technologies

Features:

- Temperature-responsive
- pH-sensitive
- Mucoadhesive

3. Manufacturing Considerations

A. Nasal Preparations

Table 7: Manufacturing Parameters

Process	**Control**	**Specification**
Filtration	Pore size	0.22 μm
Filling	Volume	±2%
Sterilization	Method	Aseptic/Terminal

B. Ear Preparations

Critical factors:

- Particle size control
- Viscosity adjustment
- Sterility maintenance

4. Quality Control

Table 8: Quality Parameters

Test	Method	Specification
Spray pattern	Laser diffraction	Product-specific
Droplet size	Dynamic analysis	20-120 μm
Content uniformity	HPLC/UV	90-110%

5. Advanced Features

A. Nasal Devices

Table 9: Device Technologies

Type	Feature	Application
Unit dose	Precise delivery	Systemic drugs
Bi-directional	Enhanced distribution	Vaccines
Electronic	Smart delivery	Controlled dosing

B. Ear Delivery Systems

Innovations:

- Controlled flow
- Temperature indication
- pH monitoring

6. Absorption Enhancement

Table 10: Enhancer Technologies

Approach	Mechanism	Example
Surfactants	Membrane modification	Polysorbates
Chelators	Tight junction opening	EDTA
Enzyme inhibitors	Metabolic protection	Peptidase inhibitors

7. Stability Considerations

A. Environmental Factors

Table 11: Stability Parameters

Factor	Control	Method
Temperature	2-8°C/25°C	Controlled storage
Light	Protection	Amber containers
Humidity	Control	Packaging

8. Special Formulations

A. Pediatric Preparations

Requirements:

- Age-appropriate doses
- Safe preservatives
- Easy administration

B. Modified Release Systems

Table 12: Release Technologies

System	Mechanism	Application
Matrix	Diffusion control	Extended release
In-situ gel	Temperature/pH triggered	Prolonged contact
Intelligent systems	Responsive release	Smart delivery

9. Safety Considerations

Key Aspects:

- Local irritation
- Systemic absorption
- Preservative safety

Table 13: Safety Parameters

Parameter	Test	Requirement
Irritation	Animal studies	Non-irritant
Toxicity	Safety studies	Within limits
Sterility	USP methods	Sterile

10. Future Trends

Emerging Technologies:

- 3D printed devices
- Smart delivery systems
- Biosensors
- Personalized formulations

Table 14: Future Developments

Technology	**Feature**	**Benefit**
Smart sensors	Monitoring	Better compliance
Bioprinting	Custom devices	Patient-specific
AI integration	Dose optimization	Enhanced efficacy

These advanced aspects of nasal and ear preparations demonstrate the complexity and sophistication of modern formulation approaches, aimed at optimizing drug delivery while ensuring product safety and efficacy.

Summary

Nasal and ear preparations are specialized dosage forms designed for administration to the nasal cavity and ear canal, respectively. These routes offer advantages in terms of local drug delivery and, in the case of nasal preparations, potential for systemic absorption bypassing first-pass metabolism. Nasal preparations include solutions, suspensions, gels, and powders for intranasal administration. These formulations are designed to deliver drugs for local effects (e.g., decongestants, antihistamines) or systemic absorption (e.g., migraine treatments, vaccines). Key considerations in nasal formulations include tonicity, pH, and viscosity to ensure compatibility with nasal mucosa and minimize irritation. Mucoadhesive polymers may be incorporated to prolong residence time and enhance drug absorption. Ear preparations, primarily solutions and suspensions, are formulated for treating conditions of the external ear canal. These preparations must be sterile if intended for use in cases of perforated eardrums. Formulation challenges include ensuring appropriate viscosity for easy administration and retention in the ear canal, and maintaining stability in the presence of cerumen (ear wax). For both nasal and ear preparations, selection of preservatives is critical, balancing antimicrobial efficacy with minimal irritation to sensitive tissues. Manufacturing processes for these preparations typically involve aseptic processing techniques, particularly for sterile products. Specialized filling equipment is used to ensure accurate dosing in unit-dose containers or metered-dose spray devices. Quality control measures include tests for sterility, particulate matter, spray pattern (for nasal sprays), and dose uniformity. Stability testing considers factors like drug degradation, microbial contamination, and compatibility with packaging materials. Challenges in developing nasal and ear preparations include achieving consistent and accurate dosing, ensuring adequate drug solubility and stability, and minimizing systemic absorption for locally acting drugs. Novel approaches in these areas include the development of temperature-sensitive gels for improved retention, nanoparticle-based delivery systems for enhanced penetration, and the use of cyclodextrins to improve drug solubility and stability.

Multiple Choice Questions

1. Which of the following is NOT a type of nasal preparation?
   a) Nasal spray
   b) Nasal gel
   c) Nasal powder
   d) Nasal tablet
2. What is the primary advantage of nasal drug delivery over oral administration?
   a) Higher drug loading capacity
   b) Avoidance of first-pass metabolism
   c) Longer duration of action
   d) Lower production cost
3. Which of the following excipients is commonly used as a preservative in nasal preparations?
   a) Benzalkonium chloride
   b) Sodium chloride
   c) Propylene glycol
   d) Methylcellulose
4. The term "mucociliary clearance" in nasal drug delivery refers to:
   a) The process of drug absorption through nasal mucosa
   b) The removal of particles from the nasal cavity by ciliary movement
   c) The breaking down of the drug in nasal secretions
   d) The irritation of nasal mucosa by the drug
5. Which type of nasal preparation is most suitable for systemic drug delivery?
   a) Nasal ointment
   b) Nasal powder
   c) Nasal spray
   d) Nasal gel

6. What is the primary purpose of an isotonicity agent?
   a) To improve drug solubility
   b) To prevent microbial growth
   c) To match the osmotic pressure of nasal secretions
   d) To enhance drug absorption
7. Which of the following factors does NOT affect drug absorption through the nasal mucosa?
   a) Molecular weight of the drug
   b) pH of the formulation
   c) Viscosity of the formulation
   d) Color of the formulation
8. The term "rhinorrhea" in nasal drug delivery refers:
   a) Nasal congestion
   b) Excessive nasal discharge
   c) Nasal dryness
   d) Nasal irritation
9. Which type of ear preparation is most suitable for treating outer ear infections?
   a) Ear drops
   b) Ear ointment
   c) Ear powder
   d) Ear wash
10. What is the primary purpose of adding a surfactant to a nasal spray formulation?
    a) To improve drug solubility
    b) To reduce surface tension and improve spreading
    c) To prevent microbial growth
    d) To enhance drug absorption
11. Which of the following is an example of a mucoadhesive polymer used in nasal preparations?
    a) Propylene glycol
    b) Sodium chloride

c) Chitosan
d) Benzalkonium chloride

12. The term "otalgia" in ear preparations refers to:
    a) Ear discharge
    b) Ear pain
    c) Ear itching
    d) Ear infection
13. What is the primary purpose of adding a vasoconstrictor to a nasal decongestant spray?
    a) To improve drug solubility
    b) To reduce nasal secretions and congestion
    c) To enhance drug absorption
    d) To prevent microbial growth
14. Which of the following is NOT a common method for enhancing drug absorption through the nasal mucosa?
    a) Using penetration enhancers
    b) Increasing formulation viscosity
    c) Using mucoadhesive polymers
    d) Centrifugation
15. The term "cerumen" in ear preparations refers to:
    a) Ear wax
    b) Ear infection
    c) Ear drum
    d) Ear canal
16. Which type of nasal preparation is most suitable for local treatment of nasal allergies?
    a) Nasal ointment
    b) Nasal spray
    c) Nasal powder
    d) Nasal gel
17. What is the primary purpose of adding a buffer to a nasal or ear preparation?
    a) To improve spreadability
    b) To maintain pH stability

c) To increase viscosity
d) To enhance drug penetration

18. Which of the following factors can contribute to the irritation of nasal mucosa?
a) Isotonic formulation
b) Neutral pH
c) High concentration of preservatives
d) Low drug concentration

19. The term "tympanic membrane" in ear anatomy refers to:
a) Ear canal
b) Ear drum
c) Middle ear
d) Inner ear

20. Which of the following is an advantage of using a nasal gel over a nasal spray?
a) Faster onset of action
b) Higher dose accuracy
c) Longer contact time with nasal mucosa
d) Easier administration.

List of Important Questions

1. What are the advantages of nasal drug delivery compared to other routes of administration?
2. Describe the different types of nasal preparations used in pharmaceuticals.
3. What are the key factors affecting drug absorption in the nasal cavity?
4. How do solutions differ from suspensions in nasal formulations?
5. Explain the importance of tonicity in nasal and ear preparations.
6. What are the common preservatives used in nasal and ear formulations, and how are they selected?
7. Describe the process of formulating a stable nasal spray.
8. How is the viscosity of nasal and ear preparations controlled, and why is it important?
9. What are the challenges in formulating poorly water-soluble drugs for nasal delivery?
10. Explain the concept of mucociliary clearance and its impact on nasal drug delivery.
11. How do ear drops differ from nasal preparations in terms of formulation considerations?
12. Describe the quality control tests performed on nasal and ear preparations.
13. What are the factors affecting the stability of nasal and ear formulations?
14. How does packaging affect the sterility and shelf life of nasal and ear preparations?
15. What are the latest innovations in nasal and ear preparation technology for improving drug delivery and patient compliance?

Bibliography

1. Ugwoke MI, Agu RU, Verbeke N, Kinget R. Nasal mucoadhesive drug delivery: background, applications, trends and future perspectives. Adv Drug Deliv Rev. 2005;57(11):1640-65.
2. Illum L. Nasal drug delivery—possibilities, problems and solutions. J Control Release. 2003;87(1-3):187-98.
3. Costantino HR, Illum L, Brandt G, Johnson PH, Quay SC. Intranasal delivery: physicochemical and therapeutic aspects. Int J Pharm. 2007;337(1-2):1-24.
4. Mygind N, Dahl R. Anatomy, physiology and function of the nasal cavities in health and disease. Adv Drug Deliv Rev. 1998;29(1-2):3-12.
5. Roland PS, Rutka JA, editors. Ototoxicity. Hamilton: BC Decker; 2004.
6. Merkus P, Ebbens FA, Muller B, Fokkens WJ. The 'best method' of topical nasal drug delivery: comparison of seven techniques. Rhinology. 2006;44(2):102-7.
7. Lochhead JJ, Thorne RG. Intranasal delivery of biologics to the central nervous system. Adv Drug Deliv Rev. 2012;64(7):614-28.
8. Dhuria SV, Hanson LR, Frey WH 2nd. Intranasal delivery to the central nervous system: mechanisms and experimental considerations. J Pharm Sci. 2010;99(4):1654-73.
9. Roland PS, Marple BF, editors. Allergic rhinitis. Philadelphia: Lippincott Williams & Wilkins; 2002.
10. Ghadiri M, Chrzanowski W, Rohanizadeh R. Biomedical applications of cationic clay minerals. RSC Adv. 2015;5(37):29467-81.

CHAPTER 16

POWDERS AND GRANULES

Author

Mr. Nadeem Hasan
Associate Professor, Dept. of Pharmaceutics,
MAM College of Pharmacy, Kalaburagi,
Karnataka, India

Abstract

Powders and granules are fundamental pharmaceutical forms used both as final dosage forms and as intermediates in the production of other solid dosage forms. This section explores the properties of powders, including particle size, shape, and surface area, and their impact on powder behavior and processing. Various methods of powder production, such as comminution and precipitation, are discussed. The principles of granulation, including wet and dry granulation techniques, are examined in detail, highlighting their role in improving powder flow properties and compressibility. Factors affecting granulation processes, such as binder selection, moisture content, and process parameters, are explored. The concept of particle size distribution and its measurement techniques are addressed. Quality control tests specific to powders and granules, including flow properties, bulk density, and moisture content determination, are detailed. Special considerations for effervescent granules and powder for reconstitution are discussed. The applications of powders and granules in various pharmaceutical dosage forms, including tablets, capsules, and sachets, are highlighted.

Keywords: *Particle characteristics, Flowability, Granulation, Size distribution, Compressibility, Process optimization*

Learning Objectives

After completion of the chapter, the student should be able to:

- Define pharmaceutical powders and granules and their applications.
- Explain the properties of powders that affect their pharmaceutical use.
- Describe various methods of granulation and their significance.
- Discuss the equipment used in powder mixing and granulation processes.
- Outline the quality control tests for powders and granules.
- Analyze the factors affecting flow properties and compressibility of powders.
- Evaluate the role of powders and granules in solid dosage form development.

Powders and granules represent fundamental pharmaceutical forms essential in drug formulation and manufacturing. Understanding their properties and behavior is crucial for developing effective pharmaceutical products.

1. Fundamental Properties of Powders

A. Physical Characteristics

Table 1: Basic Powder Properties

Property	**Description**	**Significance**
Particle size	Dimensional measurement	Flow, mixing
Shape	Morphological feature	Packing, flow

Property	Description	Significance
Surface area	Available contact area	Dissolution
Density	Mass per volume	Processing

B. Flow Properties

Table 2: Flow Parameters

Parameter	Method	Acceptable Range
Angle of repose	Fixed funnel	25-40°
Carr's Index	Density ratio	<25%
Hausner ratio	Density ratio	<1.25

2. Powder Production Methods

A. Size Reduction Techniques

Table 3: Comminution Methods

Method	Equipment	Application
Milling	Ball mill	Fine powders
Grinding	Hammer mill	Coarse reduction
Micronization	Jet mill	Ultra-fine particles

3. Granulation Processes

A. Wet Granulation

Steps:

- Mixing
- Wet massing
- Screening
- Drying
- Sizing

Table 4: Wet Granulation Parameters

Parameter	Control Range	Impact
Binder concentration	2-10%	Granule strength
Moisture content	1-4%	Processing
Mixing time	Process-specific	Uniformity

B. Dry Granulation

Methods:

- Slugging
- Roller compaction

4. Process Equipment

Table 5: Granulation Equipment

Equipment	Function	Application
High shear mixer	Wet granulation	Dense granules
Fluid bed	Granulation/Drying	Porous granules
Roller compactor	Dry granulation	Direct compression

Advanced Concepts

1. Particle Engineering

Table 6: Particle Modification

Technique	Purpose	Result
Surface coating	Flow enhancement	Better processing
Crystal modification	Solubility	Improved dissolution
Agglomeration	Size control	Better flow

2. Process Control

A. Critical Parameters

Table 7: Process Controls

Parameter	Method	Specification
Moisture	LOD/KF	Product-specific
Size distribution	Sieve analysis	Target range
Bulk density	USP method	Formula-specific

3. Quality Assessment

Table 8: Quality Tests

Test	Method	Acceptance
Content uniformity	Assay	85-115%
Flow rate	Flowmeter	Product-specific

Test	Method	Acceptance
Particle size	Laser diffraction	Target range

4. Special Types

A. Effervescent Granules

Components:

- Acid source
- Base source
- Active ingredient

Table 9: Effervescent Systems

Component	Example	Function
Acid	Citric acid	Reactant
Base	Sodium bicarbonate	Reactant
Stabilizer	PVP	Moisture protection

5. Advanced Processing

A. Continuous Manufacturing

Table 10: Continuous Process Parameters

Parameter	Control	Advantage
Feed rate	Automated	Consistency
NIR monitoring	Real-time	Quality control
PAT tools	In-line	Process optimization

6. Stability Considerations

Table 11: Stability Factors

Factor	Control	Method
Moisture	Packaging	Desiccants
Temperature	Storage	Controlled conditions
Light	Protection	Appropriate packaging

7. Novel Applications

A. Modified Release Systems

Table 12: Release Technologies

Type	Mechanism	Application
Matrix	Diffusion	Sustained release

Type	Mechanism	Application
Coated	Barrier	Delayed release
Multi-unit	Multiple release	Pulsatile delivery

8. Process Optimization

Key Aspects:

- Material attributes
- Process parameters
- Equipment selection

Table 13: Optimization Parameters

Parameter	Control Method	Impact
Speed	RPM control	Granule size
Time	Process monitoring	Uniformity
Temperature	Thermal control	Moisture

9. Advanced Characterization

Table 14: Analysis Methods

Technique	Parameter	Application
Dynamic imaging	Shape analysis	Morphology
XRD	Crystal structure	Solid state
Surface analysis	Texture	Flow properties

10. Future Trends

Emerging Technologies:

- AI-driven process control
- 3D printed powders
- Smart materials
- Continuous processing

Table 15: Future Developments

Technology	Feature	Benefit
AI control	Process optimization	Better quality
3D printing	Custom particles	Specific properties
Smart systems	Responsive materials	Enhanced performance

These advanced aspects of powder and granule technology demonstrate the complexity and sophistication of modern pharmaceutical processing, aimed at producing high-quality products while ensuring efficiency and consistency in manufacturing.

The continuous development in powder and granulation technology, coupled with advanced process controls and characterization methods, enables the production of increasingly sophisticated pharmaceutical products with enhanced performance characteristics.

Summary

Powders and granules are fundamental forms in pharmaceutical manufacturing, serving both as intermediates in the production of other dosage forms and as final products. Powders consist of finely divided solid particles, while granules are aggregates of powder particles. These forms offer advantages in terms of stability, dose flexibility, and ease of handling. Powder properties, including particle size distribution, flowability, and compressibility, significantly influence their behavior during processing and their performance in final dosage forms. Granulation processes, both wet and dry, are employed to improve flow properties, reduce dust, prevent segregation, and enhance compressibility. Wet granulation involves the addition of a liquid binder to powders, followed by drying and sizing. Methods include high-shear mixing, fluid bed granulation, and extrusion-spheronization. Dry granulation, using roller compaction or slugging, is suitable for moisture-sensitive materials. Particle engineering techniques, such as spray drying and supercritical fluid technology, are used to produce powders with specific characteristics. Quality control of powders and granules involves tests for particle size distribution, bulk and tapped density, flow properties, and moisture content. Content uniformity is crucial, especially for low-dose drugs. Stability considerations include protection from moisture and potential chemical interactions between components. Manufacturing challenges include maintaining consistent particle size distribution, preventing segregation in multi-component systems, and controlling dust during handling. Novel applications of powders and granules include their use in advanced drug delivery systems, such as orally disintegrating tablets and modified-release formulations. The development of co-processed excipients, combining multiple functionalities, has expanded the capabilities of direct compression processes. Process analytical technology (PAT) is increasingly applied to monitor and control granulation processes in real-time, ensuring consistent product quality.

Multiple Choice Questions

1. Which of the following is NOT a type of pharmaceutical powder?
   a) Dusting powder
   b) Effervescent powder
   c) Divided powder
   d) Liquid powder
2. What is the primary advantage of granules over powders?
   a) Higher drug loading capacity
   b) Improved flow properties
   c) Lower production cost
   d) Better taste masking
3. Which of the following methods is commonly used for granulation?
   a) Wet granulation
   b) Dry granulation
   c) Melt granulation
   d) All of the above
4. The term "hygroscopicity" in powders refers to:
   a) The ability to absorb moisture from the air
   b) The ability to flow freely
   c) The ability to dissolve in water
   d) The ability to form a compact mass
5. Which type of powder is most suitable for direct compression into tablets?
   a) Coarse powder
   b) Fine powder
   c) Micronized powder
   d) Granulated powder
6. What is the primary purpose of adding a glidant to a powder formulation?
   a) To improve flow properties
   b) To increase particle size

c) To enhance drug dissolution
d) To prevent microbial growth

7. Which of the following factors does NOT affect the flow properties of powders?
a) Particle size
b) Particle shape
c) Moisture content
d) Color of the powder

8. The term "angle of repose" in powder characterization refers to:
a) The angle at which powder starts to flow
b) The angle formed by a heap of powder with the horizontal plane
c) The angle at which powder compresses
d) The angle between individual powder particles

9. Which type of granulation process is most suitable for heat-sensitive drugs?
a) Wet granulation
b) Dry granulation
c) Melt granulation
d) Steam granulation

10. What is the primary purpose of adding a disintegrant to a granule formulation?
a) To improve flow properties
b) To facilitate rapid breaking of granules in water
c) To increase particle size
d) To prevent microbial growth

11. Which of the following is an example of a natural glidant used in powder formulations?
a) Talc
b) Colloidal silicon dioxide
c) Magnesium stearate
d) Starch

12. The term "bulk density" in powder characterization refers to:
    a) The density of individual particles
    b) The density of the powder including inter-particle voids
    c) The density of the powder after compression
    d) The density of the powder in a liquid medium
13. What is the primary purpose of adding a binder in wet granulation?
    a) To improve flow properties
    b) To facilitate particle size reduction
    c) To hold particles together in granules
    d) To prevent microbial growth
14. Which of the following is NOT a common method for powder size reduction?
    a) Milling
    b) Grinding
    c) Trituration
    d) Fermentation
15. The term "slugging" in dry granulation refers to:
    a) The formation of large, flat compacts
    b) The separation of fine particles
    c) The addition of a liquid binder
    d) The process of sieving
16. Which type of powder is most suitable for inhalation delivery?
    a) Coarse powder
    b) Fine powder
    c) Micronized powder
    d) Granulated powder
17. What is the primary purpose of adding an anti-adherent to a powder formulation?

a) To improve flow properties
b) To prevent sticking to punch faces and die walls
c) To increase particle size
d) To enhance drug dissolution

18. Which of the following factors can contribute to powder segregation?
    a) Uniform particle size
    b) Spherical particle shape
    c) Differences in particle density
    d) Low moisture content
19. The term "fluidized bed granulation" refers to:
    a) A type of wet granulation process
    b) A type of dry granulation process
    c) A method of powder characterization
    d) A method of powder storage
20. Which of the following is an advantage of using effervescent powders over conventional tablets?
    a) Higher drug loading capacity
    b) Better taste masking
    c) Faster disintegration and dissolution
    d) Longer shelf life

List of Important Questions

1. What are pharmaceutical powders and granules, and what are their advantages as dosage forms?
2. Describe the different types of pharmaceutical powders and granules.
3. What are the key factors affecting the flow properties of powders?
4. How does particle size distribution affect the performance of powders and granules?
5. Explain the importance of bulk density and tapped density in powder formulations.
6. What are the common methods used for granulation, and how do they differ?
7. Describe the process of wet granulation and its advantages.
8. How does dry granulation differ from wet granulation, and when is it preferred?
9. What are the challenges in formulating hygroscopic powders?
10. Explain the concept of angle of repose and its significance in powder characterization.
11. How do effervescent granules work, and what are their applications?
12. Describe the quality control tests performed on powders and granules.
13. What are the factors affecting the stability of powder and granule formulations?
14. How does packaging affect the moisture content and shelf life of powders and granules?
15. What are the latest innovations in powder and granule technology for improving drug delivery and manufacturing efficiency?

Bibliography

1. Augsburger LL, Hoag SW, editors. Pharmaceutical dosage forms: tablets. 3rd ed. New York: Informa Healthcare; 2008.
2. Summers MP, Aulton ME. Granulation. In: Aulton ME, editor. Pharmaceutics: the science of dosage form design. 2nd ed. Edinburgh: Churchill Livingstone; 2002. p. 364-78.
3. Parikh DM, editor. Handbook of pharmaceutical granulation technology. 3rd ed. Boca Raton: CRC Press; 2010.
4. Schæfer T, Mathiesen C. Melt pelletization in a high shear mixer. IX. Effects of binder particle size. Int J Pharm. 1996;139(1-2):139-48.
5. Iveson SM, Litster JD, Hapgood K, Ennis BJ. Nucleation, growth and breakage phenomena in agitated wet granulation processes: a review. Powder Technol. 2001;117(1-2):3-39.
6. Tardos GI, Khan MI, Mort PR. Critical parameters and limiting conditions in binder granulation of fine powders. Powder Technol. 1997;94(3):245-58.
7. Litster J, Ennis B. The science and engineering of granulation processes. Dordrecht: Kluwer Academic Publishers; 2004.
8. Geldart D, Abdullah EC, Hassanpour A, Nwoke LC, Wouters I. Characterization of powder flowability using measurement of angle of repose. China Particuology. 2006;4(3-4):104-7.
9. Staniforth JN, Aulton ME. Powder flow. In: Aulton ME, editor. Aulton's pharmaceutics: the design and manufacture of medicines. 3rd ed. Edinburgh: Churchill Livingstone; 2007. p. 168-79.
10. Ennis BJ. Theory of granulation: an engineering perspective. In: Parikh DM, editor. Handbook of pharmaceutical granulation technology. 2nd ed. Boca Raton: Taylor & Francis; 2005. p. 7-78.

CHAPTER 17

STERILE FORMULATIONS

Author

Mrs. Jyoti Phogat

Assistant Professor, R. J. World College of Pharmacy Education and Technology, Jakhod, Rajasthan, India

Abstract

Sterile formulations are critical pharmaceutical products designed to be free from viable microorganisms, essential for parenteral administration and other applications requiring absolute sterility. This section covers various types of sterile products, including injections, ophthalmics, and large volume parenterals. The principles of sterilization, including terminal sterilization and aseptic processing, are examined in detail. Formulation considerations for sterile products, such as tonicity adjustment, pH control, and the use of preservatives in multi-dose formulations, are discussed. The manufacturing process for sterile products, including aseptic filling and lyophilization, is explored with emphasis on contamination control and validation. Clean room design and operation, including air classification and personnel gowning procedures, are addressed. Quality control measures specific to sterile formulations, such as sterility testing, endotoxin testing, and particulate matter analysis, are detailed. The challenges in developing and manufacturing sterile products, including stability issues and container-closure integrity, are discussed along with strategies to overcome them. Regulatory requirements and guidelines for sterile product manufacturing, including current Good Manufacturing Practices (cGMP), are highlighted to ensure compliance and product safety

Keywords: *Aseptic processing, Parenteral preparations, Clean room technology, Sterilization, Contamination control, Regulatory compliance*

Learning Objectives

After completion of the chapter, the student should be able to:

- Define sterile formulations and explain their importance in healthcare.
- Describe different types of parenteral preparations and their applications.
- Explain the principles of aseptic processing and sterilization methods.
- Discuss the formulation considerations for injectable products.
- Outline the manufacturing processes for different types of sterile formulations.
- Describe the quality control tests and regulatory requirements for sterile products.
- Analyze the challenges in maintaining sterility throughout the product lifecycle.

Sterile formulations represent a critical category of pharmaceutical products that must be free from viable microorganisms. These preparations are essential for parenteral administration and applications where sterility is paramount for patient safety.

I. FUNDAMENTALS OF STERILE PRODUCTS

1. Classification of Sterile Preparations

Table 1: Types of Sterile Products

Category	**Examples**	**Administration Route**
Small Volume Parenterals	Injections	IM, IV, SC
Large Volume Parenterals	Infusions	IV
Ophthalmic	Eye drops	Ocular

Category	Examples	Administration Route
Products		
Irrigation Solutions	Rinse solutions	External

2. Basic Requirements

A. Critical Parameters

Table 2: Essential Requirements

Parameter	Specification	Importance
Sterility	No growth	Patient safety
Endotoxins	<0.25 EU/mL	Pyrogenicity
Particulates	USP limits	Safety
pH	Product-specific	Stability

II. STERILIZATION METHODS

1. Terminal Sterilization

Table 3: Sterilization Techniques

Method	Parameters	Applications
Autoclave	121°C, 15 psi, 15 min	Heat-stable products
Dry heat	160-170°C, 2-4 hrs	Glass, metals
Radiation	25 kGy	Heat-sensitive items
Gas	EtO, specific cycle	Medical devices

2. Filtration Sterilization

A. Filter Types

Table 4: Filtration Systems

Type	Pore Size	Application
Depth	0.22 μm	Clarification
Membrane	0.22 μm	Sterilization
Cartridge	Multiple	Process filtration

III. CLEAN ROOM TECHNOLOGY

1. Classification Systems

Table 5: Clean Room Classifications

Class	Particles/m³	Application
ISO 5	3,520	Aseptic processing
ISO 6	35,200	Component preparation
ISO 7	352,000	Secondary packaging
ISO 8	3,520,000	Support areas

2. Environmental Monitoring

Table 6: Monitoring Parameters

Parameter	Method	Frequency
Viable particles	Active air sampling	Daily
Non-viable particles	Particle counter	Continuous
Surface monitoring	Contact plates	Per batch
Personnel monitoring	Settle plates	Per session

IV. MANUFACTURING PROCESSES

1. Aseptic Processing

A. Critical Steps

Table 7: Aseptic Process Controls

Step	Control	Monitoring
Component preparation	Pre-sterilization	Bioburden
Sterilization	Validation	Biological indicators
Aseptic assembly	Environmental	Particle counts
Filling	Process simulation	Media fills

2. Lyophilization

Table 8: Lyophilization Parameters

Phase	Parameters	Control
Freezing	-40 to -50°C	Temperature profile
Primary drying	<100 mTorr	Pressure/temp

Phase	Parameters	Control
Secondary drying	25-40°C	Moisture removal

V. QUALITY CONTROL

1. Testing Requirements

Table 9: Quality Tests

Test	Method	Specification
Sterility	USP <71>	No growth
Endotoxin	LAL test	Product-specific
Particulate matter	Light obscuration	USP limits
Container integrity	Dye penetration	No leakage

2. Validation Requirements

Table 10: Validation Programs

Type	Scope	Frequency
Process	Manufacturing	Initial/Change
Cleaning	Equipment	Annual
Media fill	Aseptic process	Bi-annual
Filter	Sterilizing filtration	Per lot

VI. ADVANCED CONSIDERATIONS

1. Container Closure Systems

Table 11: Packaging Systems

Type	Material	Application
Vials	Glass/Plastic	Small volume
Ampoules	Glass	Single dose
Bags	Plastic	Large volume
Prefilled syringes	Glass/COC	Ready-to-use

2. Preservative Systems

Table 12: Preservative Selection

Agent	Concentration	Application
Benzalkonium Cl	0.01-0.02%	Multi-dose
Phenol	0.5%	Biologicals

Agent	Concentration	Application
Thiomersal	0.01%	Vaccines

3. Stability Considerations

Table 13: Stability Parameters

Factor	Control	Method
Temperature	2-8°C/25°C	Controlled storage
Light	Protection	Amber containers
Oxygen	Headspace	Nitrogen purging

4. Process Analytical Technology (PAT)

Table 14: PAT Implementation

Technology	Application	Benefit
NIR	Moisture analysis	Real-time control
RAMAN	Chemical ID	Material verification
Particle analysis	In-line monitoring	Process control

5. Advanced Manufacturing Technologies

A. Isolation Technology

Table 15: Isolation Systems

Type	Application	Advantage
RABS	Aseptic filling	Enhanced protection
Isolators	High potency	Complete isolation
Blow-fill-seal	Unit dose	Integrated process

6. Quality Management Systems

Key Elements:

- Risk assessment
- Change control
- Deviation management
- CAPA system

7. Regulatory Compliance

Table 16: Regulatory Requirements

Agency	Guideline	Focus
FDA	cGMP	Manufacturing

Agency	Guideline	Focus
EMA	Annex 1	Sterile products
WHO	GMP	Global standards

8. Future Trends

Emerging Technologies:

- Continuous manufacturing
- Single-use systems
- Advanced robotics
- AI-driven process control

Table 17: Future Developments

Technology	Feature	Benefit
Continuous process	Integrated system	Efficiency
Robotics	Automated handling	Reduced contamination
AI control	Process optimization	Enhanced quality

9. Special Considerations

A. Biotechnology Products

Requirements:

- Cold chain
- Protein stability
- Aggregation control

B. Novel Delivery Systems

Table 18: Advanced Delivery

System	Feature	Application
Long-acting	Depot formation	Extended release
Targeted	Site-specific	Enhanced efficacy
Smart systems	Responsive	Controlled delivery

10. Risk Management

Table 19: Risk Assessment

Area	Control	Mitigation
Cross-contamination	Segregation	Facility design
Microbial control	Monitoring	Environmental control
Product quality	Testing	Process control

Summary

Sterile formulations are critical in pharmaceutical manufacturing, encompassing products for parenteral administration, ophthalmic preparations, and certain inhalation products. These formulations require the highest level of purity and absence of viable microorganisms, necessitating specialized production environments and processes. Parenteral preparations include solutions, suspensions, and emulsions for injection or infusion. Formulation considerations involve ensuring appropriate tonicity, pH, and stability, as well as compatibility with packaging materials. Lyophilization (freeze-drying) is often employed for unstable compounds, producing sterile powders for reconstitution. Ophthalmic preparations, including eye drops and ointments, require sterility and must be formulated to be non-irritating to the delicate eye tissues. Manufacturing of sterile products takes place in clean rooms with controlled air quality, temperature, and humidity. Aseptic processing, where sterile components are assembled under highly controlled conditions, is used for heat-sensitive products. Terminal sterilization methods, including autoclaving, radiation, and gas sterilization, are employed where product stability allows. Filtration through sterilizing-grade filters (typically 0.2 μm pore size) is a crucial step in many sterile manufacturing processes. Quality control for sterile products includes tests for sterility, endotoxins, particulate matter, and container integrity. Stability studies must consider potential interactions with packaging materials and the impact of sterilization processes on product quality. Challenges in sterile manufacturing include maintaining aseptic conditions throughout the process, validating sterilization methods, and ensuring product stability in the absence of preservatives. Novel approaches in sterile formulations include the development of long-acting injectable formulations, the use of novel preservative systems for multi-dose preparations, and the application of barrier isolation technology in manufacturing. Regulatory requirements for sterile products are particularly stringent, with a focus on process validation, environmental monitoring, and rigorous quality management systems.

Multiple Choice Questions

1. Which of the following is NOT a method of sterilization?
   a) Autoclaving
   b) Gamma irradiation
   c) Ethylene oxide gas treatment
   d) Freeze drying
2. What is the primary advantage of aseptic processing over terminal sterilization?
   a) Lower production cost
   b) Higher sterility assurance level
   c) Suitable for heat-sensitive products
   d) Faster production time
3. Which of the following is a common preservative used in multi-dose parenteral formulations?
   a) Benzyl alcohol
   b) Sodium chloride
   c) Propylene glycol
   d) Methylcellulose
4. The term "pyrogen" in sterile formulations refers to:
   a) A type of preservative
   b) A fever-inducing substance
   c) A sterilizing agent
   d) A type of packaging material
5. Which type of filter is most commonly used for sterilization by filtration?
   a) Depth filter
   b) Membrane filter
   c) Cartridge filter
   d) Bag filter
6. What is the primary purpose of adding an isotonicity agent to a parenteral formulation?
   a) To improve drug solubility

b) To prevent microbial growth
c) To match the osmotic pressure of blood
d) To enhance drug stability

7. Which of the following factors does NOT affect the stability of a sterile formulation?
   a) pH
   b) Temperature
   c) Light exposure
   d) Container color
8. The term "laminar airflow" in aseptic processing refers to:
   a) A type of air sterilization
   b) A unidirectional flow of filtered air
   c) A method of product cooling
   d) A type of clean room ventilation
9. Which type of parenteral preparation is most suitable for large volume administration?
   a) Ampule
   b) Vial
   c) Infusion bag
   d) Prefilled syringe
10. What is the primary purpose of adding an antioxidant to a sterile formulation?
    a) To improve drug solubility
    b) To prevent oxidation of formulation components
    c) To increase viscosity
    d) To enhance drug absorption
11. Which of the following is an example of a lyophilized sterile product?
    a) Normal saline
    b) Insulin injection
    c) Freeze-dried vaccine
    d) Eye drops

12. The term "depyrogenation" in sterile manufacturing refers to:
    a) Removal of bacteria
    b) Removal of viruses
    c) Removal of endotoxins
    d) Removal of particulate matter
13. What is the primary purpose of adding a chelating agent to a parenteral formulation?
    a) To improve drug solubility
    b) To prevent metal ion-catalyzed degradation
    c) To increase viscosity
    d) To enhance drug absorption
14. Which of the following is NOT a common method for integrity testing of sterile filters?
    a) Bubble point test
    b) Diffusive flow test
    c) Pressure hold test
    d) Centrifugation test
15. The term "blow-fill-seal" in sterile manufacturing refers to:
    a) A type of sterilization method
    b) A method of aseptic filling
    c) A type of clean room classification
    d) A method of container integrity testing
16. Which type of parenteral preparation is most suitable for self-administration by patients?
    a) Ampule
    b) Vial
    c) Infusion bag
    d) Prefilled syringe
17. What is the primary purpose of adding a bulking agent to a lyophilized formulation?
    a) To improve reconstitution
    b) To prevent cake collapse during freeze-drying

c) To increase drug stability
d) To enhance drug absorption

18. Which of the following factors can contribute to particulate matter formation in sterile products?
a) Low temperature storage
b) Use of high-quality raw materials
c) Interaction between formulation components
d) Use of sterile filters

19. The term "media fill" in aseptic processing refers to:
a) A method of sterilizing culture media
b) A simulation of the aseptic manufacturing process
c) A type of growth promotion test
d) A method of validating sterilization cycles

20. Which of the following is an advantage of using plastic containers over glass for parenteral products?
a) Better chemical resistance
b) Higher transparency
c) Lower risk of breakage
d) Better barrier properties.

List of Important Questions

1. What are sterile formulations, and why are they crucial in pharmaceutical manufacturing?
2. Describe the different types of sterile preparations used in pharmaceuticals.
3. What are the key requirements for manufacturing sterile products?
4. How does aseptic processing differ from terminal sterilization?
5. Explain the importance of environmental monitoring in sterile manufacturing.
6. What are the common sterilization methods used in pharmaceutical manufacturing, and how do they work?
7. Describe the process of formulating a stable parenteral solution.
8. How is the tonicity of parenteral preparations controlled, and why is it important?
9. What are the challenges in formulating large volume parenteral products?
10. Explain the concept of pyrogens and endotoxins, and their significance in sterile formulations.
11. How do lyophilized (freeze-dried) products differ from liquid injectables in terms of formulation and stability?
12. Describe the quality control tests performed on sterile formulations.
13. What are the factors affecting the stability of sterile formulations?
14. How does packaging affect the sterility and shelf life of parenteral preparations?
15. What are the latest innovations in sterile formulation technology for improving drug delivery and patient safety?

Bibliography

1. Akers MJ. Sterile drug products: formulation, packaging, manufacturing and quality. Boca Raton: CRC Press; 2016.
2. Denyer SP, Baird RM, editors. Guide to microbiological control in pharmaceuticals and medical devices. 2nd ed. Boca Raton: CRC Press; 2007.
3. Nema S, Ludwig JD, editors. Pharmaceutical dosage forms: parenteral medications. 3rd ed. New York: Informa Healthcare; 2010.
4. Moldenhauer J. Environmental monitoring: a comprehensive handbook. Bethesda: PDA/DHI; 2005.
5. Agalloco J, Akers J, editors. Advanced aseptic processing technology. New York: Informa Healthcare; 2010.
6. Aulton ME, Taylor KMG, editors. Aulton's pharmaceutics: the design and manufacture of medicines. 5th ed. Edinburgh: Elsevier; 2018.
7. Rathore N, Rajan RS. Current perspectives on stability of protein drug products during formulation, fill and finish operations. Biotechnol Prog. 2008;24(3):504-14.
8. Hanson MA, Jiang X, Ye W, Hemingway C. Identification of stabilizing excipients for a lyophilized monoclonal antibody formulation through stability screening. J Pharm Sci. 2016;105(5):1467-75.
9. Carpenter JF, Pikal MJ, Chang BS, Randolph TW. Rational design of stable lyophilized protein formulations: some practical advice. Pharm Res. 1997;14(8):969-75.
10. Avis KE, Lieberman HA, Lachman L, editors. Pharmaceutical dosage forms: parenteral medications. 2nd ed. New York: Marcel Dekker; 1992.

CHAPTER 18

IMMUNOLOGICAL PRODUCTS

Author

Dr. Ramu Samineni

Assistant Professor, School of Pharmacy, Joy University, Vadakangulam, Tamil Nadu, India

Abstract

Immunological products represent a specialized category of pharmaceuticals designed to stimulate, suppress, or modulate the immune system. This section explores various types of immunological products, including vaccines, immunoglobulins, and monoclonal antibodies. The principles of immunology underlying these products, such as antigen-antibody interactions and immune response mechanisms, are discussed. Vaccine development and production processes, including live attenuated, inactivated, and subunit vaccines, are examined in detail. The formulation considerations for immunological products, such as adjuvant selection, stabilization, and preservation, are addressed. Manufacturing processes specific to immunological products, including cell culture techniques, purification methods, and fill-finish operations, are explored. Quality control measures for immunological products, including potency assays, identity tests, and safety evaluations, are detailed. The challenges in developing and manufacturing immunological products, such as cold chain requirements and stability issues, are discussed along with mitigation strategies. Regulatory considerations specific to immunological products, including lot release requirements and post-marketing surveillance, are highlighted. Recent advancements in immunological product development, such as DNA vaccines and therapeutic cancer vaccines, are briefly explored to provide insight into future directions in this field

Keywords: *Vaccines, Antibodies, Immunomodulation, Adjuvants, Biological manufacturing, Potency assays*

Learning Objectives

After completion of the chapter, the student should be able to:

- Define immunological products and their role in healthcare.
- Classify different types of vaccines and their mechanisms of action.
- Explain the production processes for various types of vaccines.
- Discuss the formulation considerations for immunological products.
- Describe the quality control tests specific to vaccines and immunologicals.
- Outline the storage and handling requirements for immunological products.
- Analyze the challenges in developing and manufacturing new vaccines.

I Immunological products are specialized biological preparations designed to interact with the immune system for therapeutic or prophylactic purposes. This comprehensive overview covers their development, production, and applications.

I. CLASSIFICATION OF IMMUNOLOGICAL PRODUCTS

1. Types of Products

Table 1: Major Categories

Category	**Examples**	**Function**
Vaccines	MMR, DPT	Prevention

Category	Examples	Function
Immunoglobulins	IVIG, HRIG	Passive immunity
Monoclonal antibodies	Rituximab	Targeted therapy
Cytokines	Interferons	Immunomodulation

2. Basic Immunological Principles

Table 2: Immune Response Types

Type	Mechanism	Application
Humoral	Antibody-mediated	Vaccines
Cellular	T-cell mediated	Cancer vaccines
Innate	Non-specific	Adjuvants

II. VACCINE DEVELOPMENT AND PRODUCTION

1. Types of Vaccines

Table 3: Vaccine Platforms

Type	Examples	Characteristics
Live attenuated	MMR, BCG	Replicating
Inactivated	IPV, Flu	Non-replicating
Subunit	HBV	Protein-based
Toxoid	Tetanus	Modified toxin
mRNA	COVID-19	Genetic material

2. Production Methods

A. Cell Culture-Based Production

Table 4: Cell Culture Systems

System	Application	Advantage
Vero cells	Viral vaccines	Well-characterized
CHO cells	Recombinant proteins	High yield
Embryonated eggs	Influenza vaccines	Traditional

B. Fermentation-Based Production

Table 5: Fermentation Parameters

Parameter	Control Range	Impact
Temperature	35-37°C	Growth rate
pH	6.8-7.2	Metabolism
DO2	>30%	Cell viability

III. FORMULATION CONSIDERATIONS

1. Adjuvants

Table 6: Common Adjuvants

Adjuvant	Type	Function
Alum	Mineral	Immune stimulation
MF59	Oil-in-water	Enhanced response
CpG	Oligonucleotide	TLR activation

2. Stabilizers

Table 7: Stabilization Systems

Stabilizer	Function	Example
Sugars	Lyoprotection	Sucrose
Amino acids	Protein stability	Glycine
Surfactants	Aggregation prevention	Polysorbate 80

IV. MANUFACTURING PROCESSES

1. Upstream Processing

Table 8: Production Steps

Step	Control	Monitoring
Seed preparation	Sterility	Viability
Expansion	Growth conditions	Cell density
Harvesting	Timing	Product titer

2. Downstream Processing

Table 9: Purification Methods

Method	Purpose	Example
Filtration	Clarification	Depth filtration
Chromatography	Purification	Ion exchange
UF/DF	Concentration	TFF

V. QUALITY CONTROL

1. Testing Requirements

Table 10: Quality Tests

Test	Method	Specification
Potency	In vitro/in vivo	Product-specific
Identity	ELISA/PCR	Confirmation
Safety	Animal tests	No adverse effects
Purity	Various	>95%

2. Stability Testing

Table 11: Stability Parameters

Parameter	Condition	Duration
Real-time	2-8°C	24-36 months
Accelerated	25°C	6 months

Parameter	Condition	Duration
Stress	40°C	3 months

VI. ADVANCED ASPECTS

1. Cold Chain Management

Table 12: Storage Requirements

Product Type	Temperature	Monitoring
Live vaccines	-70 to -80°C	Continuous
Protein vaccines	2-8°C	Data loggers
Freeze-dried	Room temp	Temperature indicators

2. Novel Delivery Systems

Table 13: Delivery Platforms

Platform	Feature	Advantage
Patches	Needle-free	Easy administration
Microarrays	Multiple antigens	Broad coverage
Nanoparticles	Targeted delivery	Enhanced efficacy

3. Production Technologies

Table 14: Advanced Technologies

Technology	Application	Benefit
Single-use	Production	Flexibility
Continuous processing	Manufacturing	Efficiency
PAT	Process control	Real-time monitoring

4. Regulatory Considerations

Table 15: Regulatory Requirements

Aspect	Requirement	Agency
Lot release	Testing	National authority
Clinical trials	Safety/Efficacy	FDA/EMA
Post-market	Surveillance	WHO

5. Future Trends

A. Emerging Technologies

Table 16: Innovation Areas

Area	Technology	Impact
Platform vaccines	Universal design	Rapid development
AI/ML	Process optimization	Enhanced efficiency
Personalized vaccines	Individual-specific	Better outcomes

6. Special Considerations

A. Combination Vaccines

Table 17: Combination Products

Type	Components	Advantage
Hexavalent	DPT-HepB-Hib-IPV	Fewer injections
Pentavalent	DPT-HepB-Hib	Cost-effective

B. Therapeutic Vaccines

Table 18: Therapeutic Applications

Disease	Approach	Status
Cancer	Neo-antigens	Clinical trials
Allergies	Immunotherapy	Approved

Disease	Approach	Status
Autoimmune	Tolerance induction	Research

7. Manufacturing Challenges

Table 19: Production Challenges

Challenge	Solution	Impact
Scale-up	Process optimization	Yield
Contamination	Closed systems	Quality
Consistency	Process control	Reproducibility

8. Quality Management

Key Elements:

- Risk assessment
- Validation
- Documentation
- Change control

9. Cost Considerations

Table 20: Economic Factors

Factor	Impact	Solution
Scale	Cost per dose	Optimization
Technology	Investment	Platform approach
Market	Accessibility	Tiered pricing

10. Environmental Impact

Considerations:

- Waste management
- Energy efficiency
- Sustainable practices.

Summary

Immunological products represent a complex and rapidly evolving category of pharmaceuticals, encompassing vaccines, immunoglobulins, and other biologics that interact with the immune system. These products play a crucial role in preventing and treating infectious diseases, autoimmune disorders, and certain cancers. Vaccines, which stimulate the immune system to produce antibodies against specific pathogens, can be categorized as live attenuated, inactivated, subunit, toxoid, or recombinant vaccines. Each type presents unique challenges in formulation, manufacturing, and stability. Vaccine production often involves the cultivation of microorganisms or the expression of antigens in cell cultures, followed by purification and formulation steps. Adjuvants may be added to enhance immune response. Immunoglobulins, derived from human plasma or produced through recombinant DNA technology, are used for passive immunization and treating various immune disorders. Their production involves complex purification processes to ensure safety and efficacy. Monoclonal antibodies, a key class of immunological products, are produced using hybridoma or recombinant DNA technology and are increasingly important in targeted therapies. Formulation of immunological products must consider factors such as antigen stability, adjuvant compatibility, and preservation of biological activity. Many of these products require cold chain storage and distribution. Manufacturing processes for immunological products are highly specialized, often involving bioreactors for cell culture, chromatographic purification techniques, and aseptic processing. Quality control is rigorous, including tests for potency, purity, identity, and safety. Specific assays may include in vitro antigen quantification and in vivo immunogenicity studies. Stability testing is crucial, considering factors like temperature sensitivity and potential for aggregation or degradation. Regulatory oversight for immunological products is particularly stringent, with extensive clinical trials required to demonstrate safety and efficacy. Challenges in this field include ensuring consistent production of complex biological molecules, maintaining cold chain integrity, and addressing the potential for immunogenicity of biologic drugs. Emerging technologies in immunological products include the development of DNA and mRNA vaccines, virus-like particle vaccines, and personalized cancer vaccines. The COVID-19 pandemic has accelerated innovation in vaccine technology and manufacturing, leading to rapid advances in areas like mRNA-based vaccines and novel adjuvant systems.

Multiple Choice Questions

1. Which of the following is NOT a type of immunological product?
   a) Vaccine
   b) Antiserum
   c) Immunoglobulin
   d) Antibiotic
2. What is the primary advantage of live attenuated vaccines over inactivated vaccines?
   a) Longer shelf life
   b) Stronger immune response
   c) Fewer side effects
   d) Lower production cost
3. Which of the following is a common adjuvant used in vaccine formulations?
   a) Aluminum hydroxide

b) Sodium chloride
c) Sucrose
d) Glycerin

4. The term "herd immunity" in vaccination refers to:
a) Immunity in animals
b) Immunity in a large proportion of a population
c) Immunity against multiple diseases
d) Immunity in healthcare workers

5. Which type of vaccine contains killed whole microorganisms?
a) Live attenuated vaccine
b) Inactivated vaccine
c) Subunit vaccine
d) Toxoid vaccine

6. What is the primary purpose of adding a stabilizer to a vaccine formulation?
a) To improve antigen solubility
b) To prevent microbial growth
c) To maintain antigen potency during storage
d) To enhance immune response

7. Which of the following factors does NOT affect the stability of a vaccine?
a) Temperature
b) Light exposure
c) Freeze-thaw cycles
d) Container shape

8. The term "cold chain" in vaccine distribution refers to:
a) A type of vaccine sterilization
b) A temperature-controlled supply chain
c) A method of vaccine administration
d) A type of vaccine packaging

9. Which type of immunological product is used for passive immunization?
a) Live attenuated vaccine

b) Inactivated vaccine
c) Immunoglobulin
d) Toxoid vaccine

10. What is the primary purpose of adding a preservative to a multi-dose vaccine vial?
a) To improve antigen stability
b) To prevent microbial growth
c) To enhance immune response
d) To facilitate antigen delivery

11. Which of the following is an example of a recombinant vaccine?
a) Oral polio vaccine
b) Hepatitis B vaccine
c) Whole-cell pertussis vaccine
d) Rabies vaccine

12. The term "seroconversion" in vaccine efficacy refers to:
a) The development of detectable antibodies in the blood
b) The attenuation of a live virus
c) The inactivation of a bacterial toxin
d) The conjugation of a polysaccharide antigen

13. What is the primary purpose of adding an adjuvant to a vaccine formulation?
a) To improve antigen solubility
b) To prevent microbial growth
c) To enhance and prolong immune response
d) To facilitate antigen delivery

14. Which of the following is NOT a common route of vaccine administration?
a) Intramuscular
b) Subcutaneous
c) Oral
d) Intravenous

15. The term "conjugate vaccine" refers to:
    a) A vaccine containing multiple antigens
    b) A vaccine where a weak antigen is linked to a carrier protein
    c) A vaccine produced by genetic engineering
    d) A vaccine containing inactivated toxins
16. Which type of immunological product is most suitable for providing immediate protection against tetanus?
    a) Tetanus toxoid vaccine
    b) Tetanus immunoglobulin
    c) Tetanus antiserum
    d) Tetanus live attenuated vaccine
17. What is the primary purpose of a vaccine diluent?
    a) To improve antigen stability
    b) To prevent microbial growth
    c) To reconstitute lyophilized vaccines
    d) To enhance immune response
18. Which of the following factors can contribute to reduced vaccine efficacy?
    a) Proper storage temperature
    b) Administration of the correct dose
    c) Concurrent administration of multiple vaccines
    d) Exposure to freezing temperatures during storage
19. The term "prime-boost strategy" in vaccination refers to:
    a) Administration of a high initial dose followed by lower doses
    b) Use of different types of vaccines for initial and booster doses
    c) Simultaneous administration of multiple vaccines
    d) Administration of vaccines at specific time intervals

20. Which of the following is an advantage of DNA vaccines over traditional vaccines?
    a) Easier production and storage
    b) No risk of infection
    c) Stronger immune response
    d) Lower production cost.

List of Important Questions

1. What are immunological products, and how do they differ from traditional pharmaceuticals?
2. Describe the different types of vaccines and their mechanisms of action.
3. What are the key considerations in formulating and manufacturing vaccines?
4. How do monoclonal antibodies work, and what are their therapeutic applications?
5. Explain the process of plasma fractionation and its importance in producing immunoglobulins.
6. What are the challenges in maintaining the stability of immunological products?
7. Describe the cold chain requirements for vaccine storage and distribution.
8. How are adjuvants used in vaccine formulations, and what is their purpose?
9. What are the differences between live attenuated and inactivated vaccines?
10. Explain the concept of herd immunity and its relevance to vaccination programs.
11. How are immunological products tested for potency and safety?
12. Describe the process of developing and manufacturing a new vaccine.
13. What are the regulatory considerations specific to immunological products?

14. How does the production of recombinant vaccines differ from traditional methods?
15. What are the latest innovations in immunological product development and delivery?

Bibliography

1. Robinson JR, Lee VH, editors. Controlled drug delivery: fundamentals and applications. 2nd ed. New York: Marcel Dekker; 1987.
2. Plotkin SA, Orenstein WA, Offit PA, editors. Vaccines. 6th ed. Philadelphia: Elsevier Saunders; 2013.
3. Crommelin DJA, Sindelar RD, Meibohm B, editors. Pharmaceutical biotechnology: fundamentals and applications. 5th ed. Cham: Springer; 2019.
4. Singh M, O'Hagan D. Advances in vaccine adjuvants. Nat Biotechnol. 1999;17(11):1075-81.
5. Peek LJ, Middaugh CR, Berkland C. Nanotechnology in vaccine delivery. Adv Drug Deliv Rev. 2008;60(8):915-28.
6. Klinman DM, Currie D, Gursel I, Verthelyi D. Use of CpG oligodeoxynucleotides as immune adjuvants. Immunol Rev. 2004;199:201-16.
7. O'Hagan DT, Singh M, Ulmer JB. Microparticles for the delivery of DNA vaccines. Immunol Rev. 2004;199:191-200.
8. Levine MM, Dougan G, Good MF, Liu MA, Nabel GJ, Nataro JP, et al. New generation vaccines. 4th ed. Boca Raton: CRC Press; 2010.
9. Aguilar JC, Rodríguez EG. Vaccine adjuvants revisited. Vaccine. 2007;25(19):3752-62.
10. Schijns VE. Immunological concepts of vaccine adjuvant activity. Curr Opin Immunol. 2000;12(4):456-63

CHAPTER 19

PHARMACEUTICAL MANUFACTURING PLANT

Author

Mr. Sharib Jamal
Associate Professor, Dept. of Pharmaceutics, Mesco Institute of Pharmacy, Amroha, Uttar Pradesh, India

Abstract

Pharmaceutical manufacturing plants are complex facilities designed to produce high-quality medicinal products in compliance with regulatory standards. This section provides an overview of the key components and considerations in designing and operating a pharmaceutical manufacturing plant. The layout and design principles of manufacturing facilities, including material and personnel flow, are discussed with emphasis on contamination control and operational efficiency. Various production areas, such as dispensing, granulation, compression, and packaging, are explored along with their specific equipment requirements. The concept of current Good Manufacturing Practices (cGMP) and its implementation in facility design and operation is examined. Utility systems critical to pharmaceutical manufacturing, including HVAC, water purification, and compressed air systems, are addressed. Quality assurance and quality control functions within the manufacturing plant, including in-process controls and finished product testing, are detailed. Environmental monitoring programs and their role in maintaining product quality are discussed. The importance of documentation systems, including batch records and standard operating procedures, is highlighted. Facility validation processes, including equipment qualification and process validation, are explored.

Keywords: *cGMP compliance, Facility design, Contamination control, Utilities, Process validation, Quality systems*

Learning Objectives

After completion of the chapter, the student should be able to:

- Describe the layout and design considerations for a pharmaceutical manufacturing plant.
- Explain the concept of Good Manufacturing Practices (GMP) in pharmaceutical production.
- Discuss the different zones in a pharmaceutical plant and their specific requirements.
- Outline the utilities and support systems needed in a pharmaceutical facility.
- Describe the environmental control measures in pharmaceutical manufacturing.
- Analyze the role of automation and process control in modern pharmaceutical plants.
- Evaluate the regulatory requirements for pharmaceutical manufacturing facilities.

A Pharmaceutical manufacturing plant is a specialized facility designed to produce pharmaceutical products under strictly controlled conditions to ensure product quality, safety, and regulatory compliance.

I. FACILITY DESIGN AND LAYOUT

1. Basic Design Principles

Table 1: Design Considerations

Aspect	Requirement	Purpose
Flow	Unidirectional	Cross-contamination prevention

Aspect	Requirement	Purpose
Zoning	Classification	Product protection
Segregation	Physical barriers	Containment
Access control	Airlocks	Personnel/material control

2. Manufacturing Areas

Table 2: Production Zones

Zone	Classification	Activity
Warehousing	ISO 8	Storage
Dispensing	ISO 7	Weighing
Production	ISO 7/8	Manufacturing
Sterile area	ISO 5/7	Aseptic processing

II. FACILITY REQUIREMENTS

1. Structural Elements

Table 3: Construction Requirements

Element	Specification	Purpose
Walls	Epoxy-coated	Cleanable
Floors	Seamless	Sanitizable
Ceilings	Sealed	Particle control
Doors	Interlocked	Access control

2. Utility Systems

Table 4: Critical Utilities

System	Specification	Application
HVAC	HEPA filtered	Air quality
Water	USP/WFI	Production
Compressed air	Oil-free	Process/controls
Steam	Clean/pure	Sterilization

III. PRODUCTION AREAS

1. Manufacturing Sections

Table 5: Production Departments

Department	Function	Equipment
Dispensing	Material preparation	Scales
Granulation	Intermediate processing	Mixers
Compression	Solid dosage	Tablet press
Coating	Film/sugar coating	Coating pans
Packaging	Primary/secondary	Packaging lines

2. Support Areas

Table 6: Auxiliary Facilities

Area	Function	Requirements
QC lab	Testing	Instruments
Maintenance	Equipment support	Workshop
Storage	Raw materials	Temperature control
Documentation	Records	Secure area

IV. ENVIRONMENTAL CONTROLS

1. Air Handling

Table 7: HVAC Parameters

Parameter	Requirement	Monitoring
Temperature	22±3°C	Continuous
Humidity	45±5% RH	Continuous
Pressure	Differential	Real-time
Filtration	HEPA/ULPA	Regular testing

2. Clean Room Classification

Table 8: Clean Room Standards

Class	Particles/m³	Application
ISO 5	3,520	Sterile processing
ISO 6	35,200	Critical areas
ISO 7	352,000	General production

Class	Particles/m^3	Application
ISO 8	3,520,000	Support areas

V. QUALITY SYSTEMS

1. Quality Control

Table 9: Testing Requirements

Type	Method	Frequency
Raw materials	USP/EP	Per receipt
In-process	Various	Per batch
Finished product	Comprehensive	Per batch
Stability	ICH conditions	Scheduled

2. Documentation

Table 10: Record Types

Document	Purpose	Retention
Batch records	Manufacturing	7 years
SOPs	Procedures	Current
Validation	Qualification	Life of equipment
Training	Personnel	Employment

VI. FACILITY MANAGEMENT

1. Maintenance Programs

Table 11: Maintenance Types

Type	Frequency	Scope
Preventive	Scheduled	Routine
Predictive	Monitored	Based on condition
Corrective	As needed	Repairs

2. Cleaning and Sanitization

Table 12: Cleaning Programs

Area	Method	Frequency
Production	SOP-based	Per batch
Clean rooms	Validated	Daily
Support areas	Standard	Scheduled

VII. ADVANCED SYSTEMS

1. Automation and Control

Table 13: Control Systems

System	Function	Benefit
SCADA	Monitoring	Real-time data
BMS	Building management	Efficiency
EMS	Environmental	Compliance

2. Material Handling

Table 14: Material Systems

System	Application	Feature
ASRS	Warehouse	Automated
AGVs	Transport	Unmanned
RFID	Tracking	Real-time

VIII. REGULATORY COMPLIANCE

1. GMP Requirements

Table 15: GMP Elements

Element	Requirement	Implementation
Personnel	Training	Documentation
Procedures	SOPs	Control
Process	Validation	Monitoring
Product	Testing	Release

2. Validation Requirements

Table 16: Validation Types

Type	Scope	Frequency
DQ	Design	Initial
IQ	Installation	New equipment
OQ	Operation	Setup
PQ	Performance	Process

IX. MODERN TRENDS

1. Industry 4.0 Integration

Table 17: Digital Technologies

Technology	Application	Benefit
IoT	Monitoring	Connectivity
AI/ML	Process control	Optimization
Digital twin	Simulation	Risk reduction

2. Sustainability Measures

Table 18: Green Initiatives

Initiative	Implementation	Impact
Energy	Efficient systems	Cost reduction
Water	Recycling	Conservation
Waste	Management	Environmental

X. SPECIAL CONSIDERATIONS

1. Safety Systems

Table 19: Safety Measures

System	Purpose	Implementation
Fire	Protection	Suppression
Emergency	Response	Procedures
Security	Access	Control

2. Future Adaptability

Table 20: Flexibility Features

Feature	Purpose	Benefit
Modular design	Expansion	Adaptability
Multi-purpose	Various products	Versatility
Scalable	Capacity	Growth

Summary

A pharmaceutical manufacturing plant is a complex facility designed to produce medicinal products under highly controlled conditions. The design and operation of these plants are governed by stringent regulatory requirements, including Good Manufacturing Practices (GMP). The layout of a pharmaceutical plant typically includes areas for raw material receiving and storage, production, packaging, quality control laboratories, and warehousing for finished products. Clean room technology is a crucial aspect, with different classes of clean rooms used depending on the products being manufactured and the level of environmental control required. HVAC systems play a critical role in maintaining appropriate temperature, humidity, and air quality. Water systems are another key component, providing various grades of water including purified water and water for injection. Production areas are equipped with specialized machinery for various unit operations such as mixing, granulation, tableting, and filling. Utilities such as steam, compressed air, and nitrogen are distributed throughout the facility. Material flow and personnel movement are carefully planned to minimize cross-contamination risks. Modern pharmaceutical plants increasingly incorporate automation and process analytical technology (PAT) to enhance efficiency and ensure consistent product quality. Facility design must consider containment strategies for highly potent compounds and segregation of different product types (e.g., penicillins, hormones) to prevent cross-contamination. Environmental considerations, including waste management and energy efficiency, are becoming increasingly important in plant design and operation. Validation of facilities, equipment, and processes is a critical aspect of pharmaceutical plant operation, ensuring that all systems consistently perform as intended. Challenges in pharmaceutical plant design and operation include maintaining flexibility to accommodate different product types, implementing new technologies while ensuring regulatory compliance, and managing the increasing complexity of supply chains and global operations.

Multiple Choice Questions

1. Which of the following is NOT a typical zone in a pharmaceutical manufacturing facility?
   a) Warehouse
   b) Production area
   c) Quality control laboratory
   d) Retail pharmacy
2. What is the primary purpose of HVAC systems in pharmaceutical manufacturing?
   a) To provide comfortable working conditions
   b) To control temperature, humidity, and air cleanliness
   c) To reduce energy consumption
   d) To eliminate odors
3. Which type of flow is ideal for personnel and materials in a pharmaceutical plant?
   a) Circular flow
   b) Random flow
   c) Unidirectional flow
   d) Bidirectional flow
4. What is the purpose of an airlock in a pharmaceutical manufacturing facility?
   a) To prevent air contamination between areas of different cleanliness
   b) To store air cylinders

c) To test air quality
d) To compress air for pneumatic systems

5. Which of the following is NOT a common material used for floors in pharmaceutical manufacturing areas?
   a) Epoxy resin
   b) Vinyl
   c) Carpet
   d) Polyurethane
6. What is the primary purpose of a clean room in pharmaceutical manufacturing?
   a) To store raw materials
   b) To provide a controlled environment for sensitive processes
   c) To conduct quality control tests
   d) To package finished products
7. Which of the following is NOT a typical utility system in a pharmaceutical plant?
   a) Purified water system
   b) Compressed air system
   c) Solar power system
   d) Steam generation system
8. What is the purpose of a laminar air flow unit in a pharmaceutical manufacturing area?
   a) To provide general ventilation
   b) To create a unidirectional flow of filtered air
   c) To remove odors
   d) To heat the manufacturing area
9. Which of the following is NOT a typical area in the quality control department of a pharmaceutical plant?
   a) Microbiology laboratory
   b) Instrumental analysis laboratory

c) Manufacturing area
d) Stability testing area

10. What is the primary purpose of an effluent treatment plant in a pharmaceutical facility?
    a) To treat drinking water
    b) To purify process water
    c) To treat wastewater before discharge
    d) To generate steam for manufacturing processes
11. Which of the following is a key consideration in the layout design of a pharmaceutical plant?
    a) Maximizing the use of windows for natural light
    b) Minimizing the distance between related operations
    c) Providing recreational areas for employees
    d) Incorporating decorative elements in production areas
12. What is the purpose of a pass-through box in a pharmaceutical manufacturing area?
    a) To transfer materials between areas of different cleanliness
    b) To store documents
    c) To conduct quality control tests
    d) To dispose of waste materials
13. Which of the following is NOT a typical method for room pressure control in clean rooms?
    a) Positive pressure
    b) Negative pressure
    c) Cascade pressure
    d) Atmospheric pressure
14. What is the primary purpose of a gowning area in a pharmaceutical manufacturing

facility?
a) To store clean room garments
b) To change into appropriate clean room attire
c) To conduct employee meetings
d) To perform quality control tests

15. Which of the following is NOT a common type of water used in pharmaceutical manufacturing?
a) Purified water
b) Water for injection
c) Distilled water
d) Tap water

16. What is the purpose of a high-efficiency particulate air (HEPA) filter in pharmaceutical manufacturing?
a) To remove large particles from the air
b) To remove microorganisms and fine particles from the air
c) To control humidity
d) To regulate temperature

17. Which of the following is NOT a typical consideration in the selection of construction materials for a pharmaceutical plant?
a) Ease of cleaning
b) Resistance to chemicals
c) Aesthetic appeal
d) Particle shedding properties

18. What is the primary purpose of an environmental monitoring program in a pharmaceutical manufacturing facility?
a) To control energy consumption
b) To detect and control microbial and particulate contamination

c) To regulate temperature and humidity
d) To manage waste disposal

19. Which of the following is NOT a typical area in the warehouse of a pharmaceutical plant?
    a) Raw material storage
    b) Finished product storage
    c) Quarantine area
    d) Production area
20. What is the purpose of a clean steam system in a pharmaceutical manufacturing facility?
    a) To clean equipment
    b) To sterilize equipment and materials
    c) To heat the manufacturing area
    d) To generate electricity.

List of Important Questions

1. What are the key components of a pharmaceutical manufacturing plant?
2. Describe the importance of facility design in ensuring product quality and regulatory compliance.
3. What are the main considerations in designing clean rooms for pharmaceutical manufacturing?
4. How does HVAC system design affect the quality of pharmaceutical products?
5. Explain the concept of material flow and its importance in plant layout.
6. What are the key utilities required in a pharmaceutical manufacturing plant?
7. Describe the different types of water used in pharmaceutical manufacturing and their purification methods.
8. How is cross-contamination prevented in multi-product manufacturing facilities?

9. What are the requirements for storage areas in a pharmaceutical plant?
10. Explain the importance of waste management in pharmaceutical manufacturing.
11. How does automation impact pharmaceutical manufacturing processes?
12. Describe the role of process analytical technology (PAT) in modern pharmaceutical plants.
13. What are the key considerations in designing a facility for sterile product manufacturing?
14. How do regulatory requirements influence pharmaceutical plant design and operation?
15. What are the latest trends and innovations in pharmaceutical manufacturing plant design?

Bibliography

1. Cole GC. Pharmaceutical production facilities: design and applications. 2nd ed. Boca Raton: CRC Press; 1998.
2. Signore AA, Jacobs T. Good design practices for GMP pharmaceutical facilities. 2nd ed. Boca Raton: CRC Press; 2016.
3. Agalloco J, Carleton FJ, editors. Validation of pharmaceutical processes. 3rd ed. New York: Informa Healthcare; 2008.
4. Haider SI, Asif ES. Quality control training manual: comprehensive training guide for API, finished pharmaceutical and biotechnologies laboratories. Boca Raton: CRC Press; 2011.
5. Nally JD, editor. Good manufacturing practices for pharmaceuticals. 6th ed. Boca Raton: CRC Press; 2007.
6. Baseman HS, Mollah AH. Risk management applications in pharmaceutical and biopharmaceutical manufacturing. Hoboken: John Wiley & Sons; 2013.
7. Pluta PL, Poska RP. Pharmaceutical facilities: HVAC systems design. In: Swarbrick J, editor. Encyclopedia of pharmaceutical technology. 3rd ed. New York: Informa Healthcare; 2007. p. 2771-83.
8. WHO Expert Committee on Specifications for Pharmaceutical Preparations. WHO good manufacturing practices for pharmaceutical products: main principles. WHO Technical Report Series, No. 986, Annex 2. Geneva: World Health Organization; 2014.
9. Gad SC, editor. Pharmaceutical manufacturing handbook: regulations and quality. Hoboken: John Wiley & Sons; 2008.
10. Berry IR, Nash RA, editors. Pharmaceutical process validation. 2nd ed. New York: Marcel Dekker; 1993.

CHAPTER 20

QUALITY CONTROL AND QUALITY ASSURANCE

Author

Mr. Vijaya Kumar Voleti
Assistant Professor, School of Pharmacy,
Sathyabama Institute of Science and Technology,
Chennai, Tamil Nadu, India

Abstract

Quality Control (QC) and Quality Assurance (QA) are integral components of pharmaceutical manufacturing, ensuring the consistency, safety, and efficacy of drug products. This section explores the principles and practices of QC and QA in the pharmaceutical industry. The distinction between QC and QA is clarified, with QC focusing on product testing and QA encompassing broader quality management systems. Various aspects of quality control are examined, including raw material testing, in-process controls, and finished product analysis. Analytical techniques commonly used in pharmaceutical QC, such as chromatography, spectroscopy, and dissolution testing, are discussed. The concept of specifications and their development is explored, highlighting the importance of setting appropriate acceptance criteria. Quality assurance principles, including risk management, change control, and continuous improvement, are addressed. The role of documentation in quality systems, including standard operating procedures (SOPs) and batch records, is emphasized. Good Laboratory Practices (GLP) and their application in quality control laboratories are discussed. The importance of method validation and analytical instrument qualification in ensuring reliable test results is highlighted. Quality metrics and their use in monitoring and improving manufacturing processes are explored.

Keywords: *Product testing, Specifications, Method validation, Risk* *management, Compliance, Continuous improvement*

Learning Objectives

After completion of the chapter, the student should be able to:

- Define Quality Control (QC) and Quality Assurance (QA) in pharmaceuticals.
- Explain the principles of Total Quality Management (TQM) in pharmaceutical industry.
- Describe the organization and responsibilities of QC and QA departments.
- Discuss various quality control tests for different pharmaceutical products.
- Outline the documentation requirements in pharmaceutical quality systems.
- Analyze the role of statistical process control in pharmaceutical manufacturing.
- Evaluate the impact of quality systems on product safety and efficacy.

Q Quality Assurance (QA) and and Quality Assurance (QA) are fundamental components that ensure pharmaceutical products meet established standards for safety, efficacy, and quality.

I. FUNDAMENTALS OF QUALITY SYSTEMS

1. Quality Concepts

Table 1: Quality Components

Component	Focus	Activities
QC	Testing	Product analysis
QA	Systems	Process oversight
TQM	Organization	Holistic approach

2. Quality System Elements

Table 2: System Structure

Element	Purpose	Implementation
Policy	Direction	Management
Procedures	Methods	SOPs
Records	Documentation	Evidence
Review	Assessment	Improvement

II. QUALITY CONTROL OPERATIONS

1. Testing Categories

Table 3: QC Testing Types

Type	Stage	Parameters
Raw materials	Input	Identity, purity
In-process	Manufacturing	Process controls
Finished product	Output	Specifications
Stability	Post-production	Degradation

2. Analytical Methods

Table 4: Testing Techniques

Technique	Application	Parameters
HPLC	Assay	Content
UV-Vis	Identification	Identity
Dissolution	Performance	Release
Karl Fischer	Moisture	Water content

III. QUALITY ASSURANCE SYSTEMS

1. System Components

Table 5: QA Elements

Element	Function	Tools
Documentation	Control	SOPs
Validation	Verification	Protocols
Auditing	Assessment	Checklists
Training	Competency	Programs

2. Risk Management

Table 6: Risk Assessment

Aspect	Approach	Action
Identification	Analysis	Documentation
Assessment	Evaluation	Prioritization
Control	Mitigation	Implementation
Review	Monitoring	Updates

IV. DOCUMENTATION SYSTEMS

1. Document Types

Table 7: Quality Documents

Type	Purpose	Content
SOPs	Procedures	Methods
Batch records	Manufacturing	Process details
Specifications	Standards	Limits
Reports	Results	Data

2. Record Management

Table 8: Documentation Control

Aspect	Requirement	System
Creation	Authorization	Review
Storage	Security	Archive
Access	Control	Permissions
Retention	Duration	Policy

V. ANALYTICAL QUALITY CONTROL

1. Method Validation

Table 9: Validation Parameters

Parameter	Requirement	Acceptance
Accuracy	Recovery	98-102%
Precision	RSD	≤2%
Linearity	R^2	≥0.999
Specificity	Resolution	≥2.0

2. Instrument Qualification

Table 10: Equipment Qualification

Stage	Purpose	Activities
DQ	Design	Requirements
IQ	Installation	Setup
OQ	Operation	Function
PQ	Performance	Testing

VI. STATISTICAL QUALITY CONTROL

1. Process Control

Table 11: Control Methods

Method	Application	Tools
SPC	Monitoring	Charts
Sampling	Testing	Plans
Trending	Analysis	Graphs
Capability	Assessment	Indices

2. Data Analysis

Table 12: Statistical Tools

Tool	Purpose	Application
Mean	Central tendency	Average
SD	Variation	Spread
Control limits	Boundaries	Limits
Capability	Process	Performance

VII. COMPLIANCE AND REGULATIONS

1. Regulatory Requirements

Table 13: Compliance Areas

Area	Standard	Requirements
GMP	Manufacturing	Process
GLP	Laboratory	Testing
GDP	Distribution	Storage
GCP	Clinical	Trials

2. Inspection and Audits

Table 14: Audit Types

Type	Scope	Frequency
Internal	Self	Scheduled
External	Third-party	Annual
Regulatory	Authority	Periodic
Supplier	Vendor	Risk-based

VIII. CONTINUOUS IMPROVEMENT

1. Quality Metrics

Table 15: Performance Indicators

Metric	Measure	Target
Defects	PPM	<100
OOS	Percentage	<1%
Complaints	Number	Minimize
Deviations	Frequency	Reduce

2. Improvement Tools

Table 16: Quality Tools

Tool	Purpose	Application
CAPA	Correction	Issues
Six Sigma	Improvement	Process
Lean	Efficiency	Operations
5S	Organization	Workplace

IX. MODERN APPROACHES

1. Digital Quality Systems

Table 17: Digital Tools

Tool	Function	Benefit
LIMS	Lab management	Efficiency
QMS	Quality system	Integration
EBR	Batch records	Accuracy
DMS	Documents	Control

2. Advanced Analytics

Table 18: Analytical Technologies

Technology	Application	Advantage
PAT	Process analysis	Real-time
NIR	Non-destructive	Rapid
Raman	Identification	Specific
MS	Characterization	Sensitive

X. SPECIAL CONSIDERATIONS

1. Product-Specific Requirements

Table 19: Special Controls

Product Type	Requirements	Controls
Sterile	Aseptic	Environmental
Biologics	Complex	Bioassays
Controlled	Security	Tracking
Stability	Storage	Monitoring

2. Laboratory Management

Table 20: Lab Operations

Aspect	Control	System
Samples	Tracking	LIMS
Standards	Control	Storage
Results	Review	Approval
Methods	Validation	Transfer

Summary

Quality Control (QC) and Quality Assurance (QA) are integral components of pharmaceutical manufacturing, ensuring that products meet predefined specifications and are safe, effective, and consistent. Quality Control involves the testing and analysis of raw materials, in-process materials, and finished products. This includes physical, chemical, and microbiological testing using validated analytical methods. QC laboratories are equipped with a range of analytical instruments such as HPLC, GC, mass spectrometry, and spectrophotometers. Stability testing is a crucial aspect of QC, monitoring product quality over time under various environmental conditions. Quality Assurance, on the other hand, is a broader concept encompassing all aspects of the manufacturing process that can impact product quality. This includes oversight of production processes, documentation systems, personnel training, and facility management. QA is responsible for implementing and maintaining the quality management system, conducting internal audits, and managing change control processes. The concept of Quality by Design (QbD) is increasingly being adopted, emphasizing building quality into products from the development stage rather than testing it at the end. Process Analytical Technology (PAT) is another important trend, allowing real-time monitoring and control of manufacturing processes. Both QC and QA play crucial roles in ensuring compliance with Good Manufacturing Practices (GMP) and other regulatory requirements. This includes managing deviations, out-of-specification results, and corrective and preventive actions (CAPA). Documentation is a critical aspect, with both departments responsible for maintaining accurate, complete records of all quality-related activities. Challenges in pharmaceutical quality management include keeping pace with evolving regulatory expectations, managing the quality of increasingly complex global supply chains, and implementing new technologies while maintaining compliance. The trend towards personalized medicine and advanced therapies is also presenting new challenges in quality control and assurance.

Multiple Choice Questions

1. Which of the following is NOT a typical responsibility of the Quality Control department?
   a) Raw material testing
   b) In-process testing
   c) Finished product testing
   d) Marketing of products
2. What is the primary difference between Quality Control (QC) and Quality Assurance (QA)?
   a) QC focuses on product testing, while QA focuses on overall quality systems
   b) QC is performed after production, while QA is performed before production
   c) QC is mandatory, while QA is optional
   d) QC applies to raw materials, while QA applies to finished products
3. Which of the following is an example of a destructive test in pharmaceutical quality control?
   a) Visual inspection
   b) pH measurement
   c) Tablet dissolution test
   d) Weight variation test

4. What does the term "OOS" stand for in quality control?
   a) Out of Stock
   b) Out of Specification
   c) Out of Service
   d) Out of Scope
5. Which of the following is NOT a typical component of a quality management system?
   a) Standard Operating Procedures (SOPs)
   b) Employee performance reviews
   c) Change control system
   d) Document control system
6. What is the primary purpose of a stability testing program?
   a) To determine product shelf life
   b) To improve product taste
   c) To reduce production costs
   d) To increase production speed
7. Which of the following is NOT a common quality control test for tablets?
   a) Hardness test
   b) Disintegration test
   c) Sterility test
   d) Content uniformity test
8. What is the purpose of an analytical method validation?
   a) To ensure the accuracy and reliability of analytical procedures
   b) To reduce the cost of quality control testing
   c) To increase production speed
   d) To improve product taste
9. Which of the following is NOT a typical qualification in equipment validation?
   a) Installation Qualification (IQ)
   b) Operational Qualification (OQ)

c) Performance Qualification (PQ)
d) Marketing Qualification (MQ)

10. What is the primary purpose of a corrective and preventive action (CAPA) system?
a) To improve product marketing
b) To identify and address quality issues and their root causes
c) To increase production speed
d) To reduce raw material costs

11. Which of the following is NOT a typical element of Good Manufacturing Practices (GMP)?
a) Personnel hygiene
b) Equipment maintenance
c) Product pricing strategy
d) Documentation control

12. What is the purpose of an annual product quality review?
a) To evaluate the consistency of the manufacturing process
b) To plan marketing strategies
c) To determine employee bonuses
d) To design new product packaging

13. Which of the following is an example of a microbiological test in pharmaceutical quality control?
a) Assay test
b) Dissolution test
c) Sterility test
d) Hardness test

14. What is the primary purpose of a change control system in pharmaceutical quality management?
a) To manage employee work schedules
b) To control and document changes that may

impact product quality
c) To control production costs
d) To manage inventory levels

15. Which of the following is NOT a typical responsibility of the Quality Assurance department?
a) Internal audits
b) Supplier audits
c) Product manufacturing
d) Training program management

16. What is the purpose of a certificate of analysis in pharmaceutical quality control?
a) To document the results of quality control tests for a specific batch
b) To provide marketing information about a product
c) To give instructions for product use
d) To authorize product recalls

17. Which of the following is an example of a physical test in pharmaceutical quality control?
a) Assay test
b) Particle size analysis
c) Sterility test
d) Impurity test

18. What is the primary purpose of process validation in pharmaceutical manufacturing?
a) To reduce production costs
b) To increase production speed
c) To ensure consistent production of quality products
d) To improve product marketing

19. Which of the following is NOT a typical component of a product specification?
a) Description

b) Assay limits
c) Manufacturing process details
d) Impurity limits

20. What is the purpose of trend analysis in pharmaceutical quality control?
    a) To predict future sales
    b) To identify potential quality issues before they become significant
    c) To determine product pricing
    d) To plan production schedules.

List of Important Questions

1. What is the difference between quality control (QC) and quality assurance (QA) in pharmaceuticals?
2. Describe the key elements of a pharmaceutical quality management system.
3. What is Good Manufacturing Practice (GMP), and why is it important?
4. How does quality by design (QbD) differ from traditional quality control approaches?
5. Explain the concept of validation in pharmaceutical manufacturing and its importance.
6. What are the main types of analytical techniques used in pharmaceutical quality control?
7. Describe the process of batch release in pharmaceutical manufacturing.
8. How are stability studies conducted, and why are they crucial in quality assurance?
9. What is the role of documentation in pharmaceutical quality systems?
10. Explain the concept of out-of-specification (OOS) results and how they are handled.

11. How does process analytical technology (PAT) contribute to quality control?
12. Describe the importance of supplier quality management in pharmaceutical manufacturing.
13. What are the key performance indicators (KPIs) used in pharmaceutical quality systems?
14. How do regulatory inspections impact quality control and quality assurance processes?
15. What are the latest trends and innovations in pharmaceutical quality management?

Bibliography

1. Larson E. Designing and managing quality control and quality assurance systems. In: Swarbrick J, editor. Encyclopedia of pharmaceutical technology. 3rd ed. New York: Informa Healthcare; 2007. p. 908-28.
2. Nash RA, Wachter AH, editors. Pharmaceutical process validation. 3rd ed. New York: Marcel Dekker; 2003.
3. Loftus BT, Nash RA. Pharmaceutical process validation. New York: Marcel Dekker; 1984.
4. Sharp J. Quality in the manufacture of medicines and other healthcare products. London: Pharmaceutical Press; 2000.
5. Rathore AS, Winkle H. Quality by design for biopharmaceuticals. Nat Biotechnol. 2009;27(1):26-34.
6. ICH Expert Working Group. Quality risk management Q9. Geneva: ICH Secretariat; 2005.
7. WHO Expert Committee on Specifications for Pharmaceutical Preparations. WHO good practices for pharmaceutical quality control laboratories.

WHO Technical Report Series, No. 957, Annex 1. Geneva: World Health Organization; 2010.

8. Nally JD, editor. Good manufacturing practices for pharmaceuticals. 6th ed. Boca Raton: CRC Press; 2007.
9. Haider SI. Validation standard operating procedures: a step-by-step guide for achieving compliance in the pharmaceutical, medical device, and biotech industries. 2nd ed. Boca Raton: CRC Press; 2006.
10. Agalloco J, Carleton FJ, editors. Validation of pharmaceutical processes. 3rd ed. New York: Informa Healthcare; 2008.

CHAPTER 21

Novel Drug Delivery Systems

Author

Dr. Basu Venkateswara Reddy

Professor and Head, Department of Pharmaceutics, Sri.K.V.College of Pharmacy, Chikkaballapura, Karnataka, India

Abstract

Novel Drug Delivery Systems (NDDS) represent advanced approaches to delivering pharmaceutical compounds in ways that enhance therapeutic efficacy, improve patient compliance, and reduce side effects. This section explores various innovative drug delivery technologies and their applications in modern pharmaceutical practice. Controlled release systems, including matrix tablets, reservoir devices, and osmotic systems, are examined for their ability to maintain therapeutic drug levels over extended periods. Targeted drug delivery approaches, such as nanoparticles, liposomes, and antibody-drug conjugates, are discussed in the context of improving drug specificity and reducing systemic toxicity. Transdermal delivery systems, including patches and iontophoretic devices, are explored for their potential in providing non-invasive, controlled drug administration. Pulmonary drug delivery systems, such as dry powder inhalers and metered-dose inhalers, are addressed, highlighting their importance in respiratory therapeutics. The principles of mucoadhesive drug delivery for improving gastrointestinal and nasal absorption are examined. Advanced technologies like 3D printing in pharmaceutical manufacturing and its potential for personalized medicine are briefly discussed. Challenges in developing NDDS, including formulation complexities, scale-up issues, and regulatory considerations, are addressed

Keywords: *Controlled release, Targeted delivery, Nanocarriers,*

Transdermal systems, Personalized medicine, Smart therapeutics

Learning Objectives

After completion of the chapter, the student should be able to:

- Define novel drug delivery systems and their advantages over conventional dosage forms.
- Classify different types of novel drug delivery systems and their applications.
- Explain the principles of controlled release and targeted drug delivery.
- Describe various technologies used in developing novel drug delivery systems.
- Discuss the formulation considerations for different novel delivery systems.
- Analyze the challenges in developing and manufacturing novel drug delivery systems.
- Evaluate the future trends and potential of novel drug delivery technologies.

Novel Drug Delivery Systems (NDDS) represent advanced pharmaceutical technologies designed to optimize therapeutic outcomes through improved drug delivery methods.

I. FUNDAMENTAL CONCEPTS

1. Basic Principles

Table 1: NDDS Characteristics

Characteristic	**Purpose**	**Benefit**
Controlled release	Sustained levels	Better efficacy
Targeting	Site-specific	Reduced

Characteristic	Purpose	Benefit
		toxicity
Enhanced absorption	Bioavailability	Lower dosing
Smart delivery	Response-based	Precision

2. Classification Systems

Table 2: NDDS Types

System	Mechanism	Application
Matrix	Diffusion	Oral delivery
Reservoir	Membrane	Long-acting
Particulate	Carrier-based	Targeting
Transdermal	Absorption	Non-invasive

II. CONTROLLED RELEASE SYSTEMS

1. Release Mechanisms

Table 3: Release Controls

Mechanism	Process	Examples
Diffusion	Concentration	Matrix tablets
Erosion	Degradation	Biodegradable
Osmotic	Pressure	OROS systems
Swelling	Hydration	Hydrogels

2. Design Parameters

Table 4: Design Factors

Factor	Impact	Consideration
Polymer	Release rate	Molecular weight
Drug	Solubility	Particle size
Matrix	Structure	Porosity
Environment	pH/enzymes	Stability

III. TARGETED DELIVERY SYSTEMS

1. Targeting Approaches

Table 5: Targeting Methods

Method	Strategy	Application
Passive	EPR effect	Cancer
Active	Ligand-based	Specific cells
Magnetic	External field	Local delivery
pH-sensitive	Environmental	GI targeting

2. Carrier Systems

Table 6: Drug Carriers

Carrier	Size Range	Features
Nanoparticles	1-100 nm	High surface area
Liposomes	50-500 nm	Bilayer structure
Microspheres	1-1000 μm	Matrix system
Dendrimers	1-10 nm	Branched structure

IV. TRANSDERMAL DELIVERY

1. System Components

Table 7: Patch Components

Component	Function	Examples
Backing	Protection	Polyester
Matrix	Drug reservoir	Polymers
Adhesive	Attachment	Acrylates
Liner	Protection	Release film

2. Enhancement Methods

Table 8: Permeation Enhancement

Method	Mechanism	Technology
Chemical	Penetration	Enhancers
Physical	Disruption	Microneedles
Electrical	Iontophoresis	Electric field
Ultrasound	Sonophoresis	Cavitation

V. PULMONARY DELIVERY SYSTEMS

1. Inhalation Devices

Table 9: Inhaler Types

Device	Mechanism	Application
DPI	Powder	Systemic/local
MDI	Aerosol	Respiratory
Nebulizer	Solution	Acute care
Soft mist	Fine spray	Chronic use

2. Formulation Factors

Table 10: Aerosol Properties

Property	Requirement	Impact
Size	1-5 μm	Deposition
Flow	Aerodynamic	Delivery
Stability	Storage	Shelf-life
Moisture	Protection	Performance

VI. ADVANCED TECHNOLOGIES

1. Smart Systems

Table 11: Smart Features

Feature	Function	Application
Sensors	Monitoring	Feedback
Response	Adaptation	Control
Communication	Data	Management
Automation	Delivery	Precision

2. Novel Materials

Table 12: Advanced Materials

Material	Property	Use
Hydrogels	Responsive	Control
Biomaterials	Compatible	Safety
Nanomaterials	Size/surface	Targeting
Polymers	Functional	Delivery

VII. FORMULATION CONSIDERATIONS

1. Development Factors

Table 13: Development Parameters

Parameter	Impact	Control
Stability	Shelf-life	Packaging
Compatibility	Interaction	Selection
Processing	Manufacturing	Methods
Scale-up	Production	Technology

2. Quality Parameters

Table 14: Quality Aspects

Aspect	Test	Specification
Content	Assay	90-110%
Release	Dissolution	Profile
Stability	Testing	Conditions
Sterility	When needed	Pass

VIII. REGULATORY CONSIDERATIONS

1. Requirements

Table 15: Regulatory Aspects

Aspect	Requirement	Documentation
Safety	Studies	Data
Efficacy	Trials	Results
Quality	Standards	Controls
Manufacturing	GMP	Compliance

2. Documentation

Table 16: Required Documents

Document	Purpose	Content
CMC	Chemistry	Manufacturing
IND	Clinical	Safety
NDA	Approval	Complete
DMF	Supporting	Details

IX. EMERGING TRENDS

1. New Technologies

Table 17: Innovations

Technology	Application	Advantage
3D printing	Custom	Personalized
AI/ML	Design	Optimization
Bioprinting	Tissue	Regeneration
Robotics	Manufacturing	Precision

2. Future Directions

Table 18: Future Trends

Trend	Impact	Potential
Personalization	Individual	Optimization
Integration	Systems	Efficiency
Automation	Process	Control
Sustainability	Environment	Green

X. CHALLENGES AND SOLUTIONS

1. Technical Challenges

Table 19: Technical Issues

Challenge	Impact	Solution
Stability	Storage	Technology
Scale-up	Production	Process
Cost	Economics	Efficiency
Performance	Efficacy	Design

2. Market Considerations

Table 20: Market Factors

Factor	Impact	Strategy
Cost	Access	Optimization
Competition	Market	Innovation
Acceptance	Uptake	Education
Regulations	Compliance	Planning

Summary

Novel Drug Delivery Systems (NDDS) represent advanced technologies designed to optimize the delivery of pharmaceutical compounds, enhancing their efficacy, safety, and patient compliance. These systems aim to control the rate, time, and place of drug release in the body. Controlled release systems, including matrix tablets, reservoir devices, and osmotic systems, provide sustained drug levels over extended periods. Targeted drug delivery systems use various mechanisms to concentrate drugs at specific sites in the body, reducing systemic side effects. These include liposomes, nanoparticles, and antibody-drug conjugates. Transdermal drug delivery systems, such as patches and iontophoretic devices, offer non-invasive routes for systemic drug administration. Mucoadhesive systems prolong drug contact with mucosal surfaces, enhancing local or systemic effects. Pulmonary drug delivery systems, including dry powder inhalers and nebulizers, are used for both local and systemic delivery. Implantable drug delivery systems provide long-term, controlled release of drugs, often used in hormonal therapies or pain management. Stimuli-responsive systems release drugs in response to specific physiological conditions or external stimuli. The development of NDDS involves considerations of drug physicochemical properties, pharmacokinetics, and the intended therapeutic effect. Formulation challenges include ensuring drug stability within the delivery system, achieving desired release kinetics, and maintaining biocompatibility. Manufacturing of NDDS often requires specialized technologies and equipment, such as high-pressure homogenizers for nanoparticle production or aseptic processes for long-acting injectables. Quality control of NDDS includes specialized in vitro release testing methods and often requires the development of new analytical techniques. Regulatory considerations for NDDS are complex, often requiring extensive preclinical and clinical studies to demonstrate safety and efficacy. Emerging areas in NDDS include the use of 3D printing for personalized dosage forms, the development of "smart" delivery systems that can respond to biological feedback, and the application of nanotechnology for enhanced drug targeting and cellular uptake. The integration of NDDS with digital technologies, such as sensors and mobile applications, is opening new possibilities for personalized and monitored drug delivery.

Multiple Choice Questions

1. Which of the following is NOT considered a novel drug delivery system?
   a) Liposomes
   b) Transdermal patches
   c) Nanoparticles
   d) Traditional tablets
2. What is the primary advantage of controlled release drug delivery systems?
   a) Lower production cost
   b) Improved patient compliance
   c) Faster onset of action
   d) Increased drug stability
3. Which of the following is an example of a mucoadhesive drug delivery system?
   a) Buccal patch
   b) Intravenous injection
   c) Intramuscular injection
   d) Oral tablet

4. What is the primary purpose of using nanoparticles in drug delivery?
   a) To increase drug particle size
   b) To improve drug solubility and bioavailability
   c) To reduce drug potency
   d) To increase drug toxicity
5. Which of the following is NOT a common type of transdermal drug delivery system?
   a) Matrix patch
   b) Reservoir patch
   c) Drug-in-adhesive patch
   d) Oral patch
6. What is the primary advantage of pulmonary drug delivery systems?
   a) Large surface area for absorption
   b) Slower drug absorption
   c) Increased first-pass metabolism
   d) Limited to water-soluble drugs
7. Which of the following is an example of a stimuli-responsive drug delivery system?
   a) pH-sensitive polymers
   b) Conventional tablet
   c) Standard capsule
   d) Regular oral solution
8. What is the primary purpose of using cyclodextrins in drug delivery?
   a) To decrease drug solubility
   b) To increase drug particle size
   c) To improve drug stability and solubility
   d) To reduce drug potency
9. Which of the following is NOT a common type of liposome?
   a) Unilamellar vesicle
   b) Multilamellar vesicle

c) Solid lipid nanoparticle
d) Transfersome

10. What is the primary advantage of osmotic drug delivery systems?
a) Zero-order drug release
b) Faster drug absorption
c) Increased drug metabolism
d) Limited to water-soluble drugs

11. Which of the following is an example of a targeted drug delivery system?
a) Monoclonal antibody-drug conjugate
b) Conventional tablet
c) Standard capsule
d) Regular oral solution

12. What is the primary purpose of using dendrimers in drug delivery?
a) To decrease drug solubility
b) To increase drug particle size
c) To improve drug encapsulation and targeting
d) To reduce drug potency

13. Which of the following is NOT a common type of microparticle used in drug delivery?
a) Microsphere
b) Microcapsule
c) Microemulsion
d) Microchip

14. What is the primary advantage of buccal drug delivery systems?
a) Increased first-pass metabolism
b) Avoidance of first-pass metabolism
c) Slower drug absorption
d) Limited to lipid-soluble drugs

15. Which of the following is an example of an implantable drug delivery system?

a) Oral tablet
b) Transdermal patch
c) Subcutaneous implant
d) Nasal spray

16. What is the primary purpose of using hydrogels in drug delivery?
a) To decrease drug solubility
b) To increase drug particle size
c) To provide controlled drug release
d) To reduce drug potency

17. Which of the following is NOT a common type of nanocarrier used in drug delivery?
a) Polymeric nanoparticle
b) Solid lipid nanoparticle
c) Quantum dot
d) Macroparticle

18. What is the primary advantage of iontophoretic transdermal drug delivery systems?
a) Passive drug diffusion
b) Limited to lipid-soluble drugs
c) Enhanced penetration of ionic drugs
d) Decreased skin permeability

19. Which of the following is an example of a gastroretentive drug delivery system?
a) Floating dosage form
b) Transdermal patch
c) Ocular insert
d) Pulmonary inhaler

20. What is the primary purpose of using microneedles in drug delivery?
a) To increase drug particle size
b) To improve oral bioavailability
c) To enhance transdermal drug delivery
d) To reduce drug solubility.

List of Important Questions

1. What are novel drug delivery systems, and how do they differ from conventional dosage forms?
2. Describe the different types of controlled release drug delivery systems.
3. What are the advantages and challenges of using nanoparticles in drug delivery?
4. How do liposomes work as drug carriers, and what are their applications?
5. Explain the concept of targeted drug delivery and its importance in cancer treatment.
6. What are the key considerations in developing transdermal drug delivery systems?
7. Describe the working principle of osmotic drug delivery systems.
8. How do mucoadhesive drug delivery systems enhance drug absorption?
9. What are the advantages and limitations of pulmonary drug delivery systems?
10. Explain the concept of stimuli-responsive drug delivery systems and their potential applications.
11. How do implantable drug delivery devices work, and what are their therapeutic uses?
12. Describe the role of polymers in novel drug delivery systems.
13. What are the challenges in developing and manufacturing novel drug delivery systems?
14. How do regulatory agencies evaluate novel drug delivery systems for approval?
15. What are the latest innovations and future trends in novel drug delivery systems?

Bibliography

1. Thassu D, Deleers M, Pathak Y, editors. Nanoparticulate drug delivery systems. New York: Informa Healthcare; 2007.
2. Siepmann J, Siegel RA, Rathbone MJ, editors. Fundamentals and applications of controlled release drug delivery. New York: Springer; 2012.
3. Park K, editor. Controlled drug delivery: challenges and strategies. Washington, DC: American Chemical Society; 1997.
4. Koo OMY, editor. Pharmaceutical excipients: properties, functionality, and applications in research and industry. Hoboken: John Wiley & Sons; 2017.
5. Liechty WB, Kryscio DR, Slaughter BV, Peppas NA. Polymers for drug delivery systems. Annu Rev Chem Biomol Eng. 2010;1:149-73.
6. Allen TM, Cullis PR. Drug delivery systems: entering the mainstream. Science. 2004;303(5665):1818-22.
7. Langer R. Drug delivery and targeting. Nature. 1998;392(6679 Suppl):5-10.
8. Torchilin VP. Multifunctional nanocarriers. Adv Drug Deliv Rev. 2006;58(14):1532-55.
9. Mitragotri S, Burke PA, Langer R. Overcoming the challenges in administering biopharmaceuticals: formulation and delivery strategies. Nat Rev Drug Discov. 2014;13(9):655-72.
10. Peppas NA, Bures P, Leobandung W, Ichikawa H. Hydrogels in pharmaceutical formulations. Eur J Pharm Biopharm. 2000;50(1):27-46

ANSWERS TO THE MCQS

Chapter 1
1. c)
2. b)
3. b)
4. c)
5. c)
6. c)
7. c)
8. b)
9. a)
10. d)
11. c)
12. c)
13. a)
14. c)
15. d)
16. c)
17. d)
18. b)
19. c)
20. b)

Chapter 2
1. b)
2. b)
3. a)
4. b)
5. d)
6. b)
7. a)
8. c)
9. a)
10. c)
11. c)
12. c)
13. a)
14. b)
15. c)
16. d)
17. b)
18. a)
19. c)
20. b)

Chapter 3
1. c
2. b
3. b
4. b
5. a
6. a
7. c
8. a
9. c
10. b
11. a
12. c
13. d
14. b
15. c
16. a
17. c
18. b
19. d
20. b

Chapter 4
1. b
2. a
3. b
4. c
5. a
6. b
7. b
8. b
9. a
10. c
11. a
12. b
13. a
14. c
15. a
16. b
17. a
18. a
19. a
20. c

Chapter 6

1. b
2. c
3. c
4. a
5. b
6. d
7. b
8. c
9. a
10. c
11. b
12. d
13. c
14. c

15. c
16. c
17. c
18. c
19. b
20. b

Chapter 7

1. b
2. d
3. b
4. c
5. a
6. d
7. c
8. a
9. c
10. b
11. b
12. c
13. c
14. b
15. d

Chapter 8

1. b
2. d
3. b
4. b
5. a
6. d
7. c
8. b
9. c
10. b
11. b
12. b
13. b
14. b
15. a

Chapter 9

1. b
2. d
3. b
4. c
5. b
6. d
7. b
8. b
9. c
10. b
11. c
12. c
13. c
14. b
15. d

Chapter 10

1. b
2. d
3. a
4. b
5. c
6. d
7. c
8. c
9. c
10. b
11. c
12. b
13. b
14. b
15. d
16. b
17. b
18. c
19. b
20. c

Chapter 11

1. d
2. d
3. d
4. c
5. b
6. d
7. b
8. d
9. a
10. c
11. b
12. d
13. c
14. c
15. b
16. c
17. a
18. d
19. b
20. b

Chapter 12

1. a
2. d
3. b
4. b
5. c
6. d

7. b
8. c
9. a
10. c
11. b
12. b
13. b
14. c
15. b
16. d
17. b
18. b
19. b
20. b

Chapter 13

1. d
2. b
3. b
4. b
5. a
6. b
7. d
8. a
9. b
10. b
11. a
12. a
13. b
14. d
15. b
16. c
17. b
18. c
19. b
20. c

Chapter 14

1. d
2. b
3. b
4. b
5. d
6. b
7. d
8. b
9. c
10. b
11. c
12. a
13. b
14. d
15. b
16. c
17. b
18. c
19. b
20. c

Chapter 15

1. d
2. b
3. a
4. b
5. c
6. c
7. d
8. b
9. a
10. b
11. c
12. b
13. b
14. d
15. a
16. b
17. b
18. c
19. b
20. c

Chapter 16

1. d
2. b
3. d
4. a
5. d
6. a
7. d
8. b
9. b
10. b
11. a
12. b
13. c
14. d
15. a
16. c
17. b
18. c
19. a
20. c

Chapter 17

1. d
2. c
3. a
4. b
5. b
6. c
7. d

8. b
9. c
10. b
11. c
12. c
13. b
14. d
15. b
16. d
17. b
18. c
19. b
20. c

Chapter 18
1. d
2. b
3. a
4. b
5. b
6. c
7. d
8. b
9. c
10. b
11. b
12. a
13. c
14. d
15. b
16. b
17. c
18. d
19. b
20. b

Chapter 19
1. d
2. b
3. c
4. a
5. c
6. b
7. c
8. b
9. c
10. c
11. b
12. a
13. d
14. b
15. d
16. b
17. c
18. b
19. d
20. b

Chapter 20
1. d
2. a
3. c
4. b
5. b
6. a
7. c
8. a
9. d
10. b
11. c
12. a
13. c
14. b
15. c
16. a
17. b
18. c
19. c
20. b

Chapter 21
1. d
2. b
3. a
4. b
5. d
6. a
7. a
8. c
9. c
10. a
11. a
12. c
13. d
14. b
15. c
16. c
17. d
18. c
19. a
20. c

ABOUT THE AUTHORS

Dr. SOWJANYA GURUGUBELLI

Dr. Sowjanya Gurugubelli holds a B. Pharmacy, M.Tech in Biotechnology (JNTU Hyderabad), and Ph.D in Pharmaceutical Sciences (Andhra University). An Associate Professor at Aditya Pharmacy College with over 10 years of teaching experience, she received a National Award at APTICON-2022. Dr. Sowjanya has participated in DST-funded STUTI-21, published 7 research articles, presented at various conferences, and is a reviewer for two journals. She is a lifetime member of two professional bodies.

Mrs. JHANSIPRIYA MARABATHUNI V

Mrs. Jhansipriya Marabathuni V is an Associate Professor at Bellamkonda Institute of Technology and Science, Podili, with over 13 years of teaching experience. She has published more than 20 articles in reputed journals, including Scopus and PubMed indexed publications, and holds patents. A life member of APTI & IPGA, she co-authored a book on Herbal Drug Technology published by Scientific International Publishing House.

Mrs. Marabathuni has guided more than 10 PG and 20 UG students in their research projects

Mr. PRAKASH NATHANIEL KUMAR SARELLA

Mr. Prakash Nathaniel Kumar Sarella is working as an Associate Professor at Aditya College of Pharmacy, Aditya University with over 8 years of experience in teaching and research. His expertise includes nanomedicine, liposomes, polymer therapeutics, antibody-drug conjugates, and microneedle technologies, and other innovative drug delivery solutions. He published over 40 research papers and life member of APTI and IPGA

Mrs. VINNY THERISSA MANGAM

Mrs. Vinny Therissa Mangam is an Assistant Professor working at Aditya College of Pharmacy, Aditya University with over 4 years of experience in teaching, analytical method development and validation. She published 8 research papers and lifetime member of APT and IPGA. Her expertise lies in optimizing techniques, comparing methods, and transferring procedures to enable enhanced standards in pharmaceutical analysis.

Mr. SHAIKH SAMIR KARIM KARIM

Mr. Shaikh Samir Karim completed his B. Pharmacy and M. Pharm from Shri Sureshdada Jain Institute of Pharmaceutical Education and Research, Jamner, under KBC North Maharashtra University and currently serving as Lecturer in the same college. He has published 7 research articles as a corresponding author and co-author in reputed national and international journals.

Mrs. CHOLLANGI BHARGHAVI

Mrs. Chollangi Bharghavi is an Assistant Professor in the Department of Pharmaceutics at Ranchi College of Pharmacy, Ranchi. She has 3 and a half years of teaching experience and her goal is to equip pharmacy students with necessary skills for a successful career.

Mrs. PRATHYUSHA VUDDANDA

Mrs. Prathyusha Vuddanda is an Assistant Professor working at Narayana Pharmacy College, Nellore. With her expertise in pharmaceutical sciences, she contributes to the academic growth and development of pharmacy students. She is dedicated to enhancing the quality of pharmacy education and research at the institution.

Dr. BALA VENKATA SIVARAM NALLAMOLU

Dr. Bala Venkata Sivaram Nallamolu is a passionate pharmacy academician with 27 years of experience. He is currently working as Professor and HOD in the Department of Pharmaceutics at Sir CRR College of Pharmaceutical Sciences, Eluru, AP, India. Dr. Nallamolu has served for more than a decade internationally.

Mrs. VIJAYALAKSHMI M K

Mrs. Vijayalakshmi M.K. is working as an Associate Professor in department of Pharmaceutical Chemistry /Analysis at Faculty of Pharmacy, Bharath Institute of

Higher Education and Research. She has completed her post-graduation in Pharmaceutical Chemistry in Madaras Medical College, Chennai. She has vast experience in Research and Development in various industries and Organisation. Her present interest on research in Computer Aided Drug Design with strong background in various pharmaceutical field as Quality Control Chemist, Senior Research Scientist and Academic Field. She has published numerous research articles in peer reviewed national and international journals, edited book chapters and associated as an editor for many books.

Mr. ANILKUMAR VADAGA

Mr. Anil Kumar Vadaga is an esteemed Associate Professor within the department of Pharmaceutics at the GIET School Pharmacy, Rajahmundry. His academic journey reflects a deep-rooted passion for Pharmaceutics, marked by his unwavering commitment to the field. With his M. Pharm background, he has already acquired a strong foundation in Pharmaceutical Knowledge and principles. He also worked in the field of novel drug